Chronic Obstructive Pulmonary Disease (COPD)

-

From Causes to Control

by

VIRUTI SHIVAN

Masters in Clinical Psychology (Major)

"In books, as in life, it's not the size or looks but the content that matters."

DISCLAIMER: The information in this book is provided for general informational purposes only and is not intended as professional advice. Although every effort has been made to ensure the accuracy and completeness of the information, the author and publisher do not assume responsibility for errors, inaccuracies, omissions, inconsistencies, or the impact of future advancements or updates in technology and information. This book is not a substitute for proper training, diagnosis, treatment, or guidance from qualified professionals. Readers are encouraged to consult experts in the relevant fields and independently verify the information when necessary. Any slights of people, places, or organizations are unintentional and purely coincidental.

Introduction

Chronic Obstructive Pulmonary Disease (COPD) is a term that encapsulates a group of lung conditions characterized by persistent respiratory symptoms and airflow limitation due to airway and/or alveolar abnormalities, usually caused by significant exposure to noxious particles or gases. The journey through understanding, managing, and potentially reversing the impacts of COPD is both complex and deeply personal. This guide is designed not just as a resource but as a companion for those navigating the turbulent waters of a COPD diagnosis, whether for themselves or a loved one.

COPD: A Global Challenge

COPD stands as a silent epidemic, affecting millions worldwide, with numbers only predicted to rise due to increasing pollution levels and tobacco usage. It's a condition that bridges gaps across age, geography, and socioeconomic status, making it a global challenge that calls for a united front in healthcare education, policy, and research. The objective of this book is to demystify COPD, breaking down the latest in medical research and therapeutic strategies into actionable insights.

From Causes to Control

Understanding COPD begins with its causes—from the inhalation of cigarette smoke to long-term exposure to occupational dust and chemicals. This book delves into the pathophysiology of COPD, exploring how these exposures lead to the inflammation, mucus production, and eventual scarring that characterizes the disease. However, the narrative quickly shifts from the causes to focus on control, empowerment, and adaptation, ensuring that the disease does not define the individual.

Empowerment through Education

Empowerment through education is a central theme of this guide. By providing clear, comprehensive information about symptoms, diagnostic procedures, and treatment options, this book aims to demystify the disease. It emphasizes the importance of early detection and proactive management, including lifestyle modifications, pharmacotherapy, and when necessary, surgical interventions. Each section is carefully crafted to foster an understanding that can lead to actionable change, improving the quality of life for those affected.

A Personal Journey

Recognizing that COPD affects more than just the physical body, this book also addresses the psychological and social impacts. Living with COPD can be a lonely journey, marked by fear, frustration, and often, a sense of loss. Through personal anecdotes and hypothetical scenarios, readers will find stories of resilience and hope, illustrating not only the challenges but also the victories possible when navigating life with COPD.

Looking Forward

Finally, this guide doesn't shy away from looking forward. It explores the cutting-edge of COPD research, from novel pharmacological treatments to innovative surgical techniques and the promise of regenerative medicine. But it also considers the everyday—how today's decisions, from smoking cessation to air quality advocacy, can shape the future of COPD care and prevention.

In the chapters that follow, you will find a blend of scientific insight, practical advice, and personal stories, all aimed at providing a comprehensive overview of COPD. This guide is an invitation to understand, manage, and possibly even reverse the effects of COPD, paving the way for a future where the disease's impact is minimized, both for individuals and on a global scale.

Chapter 1: Understanding COPD

1.1 The Basics of Chronic Obstructive Pulmonary Disease

COPD Defined

Chronic Obstructive Pulmonary Disease (COPD) is a progressive lung disease characterized by increasing breathlessness. It encompasses two main conditions: emphysema and chronic bronchitis. Emphysema involves damage to the alveoli (air sacs) in the lungs, where gas exchange of oxygen and carbon dioxide takes place. Chronic bronchitis is defined by the presence of cough and sputum production for at least three months in each of two successive years, caused by inflammation of the lining of the bronchial tubes.

Pathophysiology

The pathophysiology of COPD involves chronic inflammation and damage to the lung tissue, particularly the smaller airways and alveoli, which lose their elastic quality. This results in air trapping and difficulty in air flow out of the lungs, leading to the characteristic symptoms of breathlessness, cough, and sputum production. Over time, the airways can thicken and become scarred, further reducing airflow. The body's attempt to repair this damage can cause mucus hypersecretion, adding to the obstruction of airflow.

Causes and Risk Factors

The primary cause of COPD is tobacco smoke, including secondhand smoke exposure. Other risk factors include exposure to air pollution, occupational dusts and chemicals, and genetic factors such as alpha-1 antitrypsin deficiency, though this is rare. The risk of developing COPD increases with age and the cumulative exposure to harmful substances.

Symptoms

The initial symptoms of COPD can be mild and often dismissed as a 'smoker's cough'. As the disease progresses, the symptoms become more pronounced and debilitating. They include:

- Persistent cough

- Increased mucus production

- Frequent respiratory infections

- Wheezing

- Shortness of breath, especially during physical activities

- Fatigue

Diagnosis

Diagnosis of COPD is primarily based on history, physical examination, and confirmation by spirometry. Spirometry is a simple test that measures how much and how quickly a person can expel air from the lungs. It helps in assessing the degree of airflow obstruction and is essential for the accurate diagnosis and staging of COPD.

Impact of COPD

The impact of COPD on an individual's life can be profound, affecting physical, emotional, and social wellbeing. Daily activities can become challenging, leading to decreased mobility and social isolation. Early diagnosis and appropriate management are critical to slowing the progression of the disease, improving quality of life, and reducing the risk of other associated conditions such as heart disease and lung cancer.

Management Overview

Management of COPD requires a comprehensive approach that includes smoking cessation, pharmacotherapy (such as bronchodilators and anti-inflammatory medications), pulmonary rehabilitation, and, in severe cases, oxygen therapy. Lifestyle modifications, including exercise and a healthy diet, play a crucial role in managing symptoms and improving the overall health status of individuals with COPD.

Understanding the basics of COPD is the first step towards empowerment and management of this condition. By recognizing the signs early and taking action, individuals can significantly impact their disease progression and quality of life.

1.2 Signs and Symptoms: Recognizing COPD

Early Recognition is Key

Recognizing the signs and symptoms of Chronic Obstructive Pulmonary Disease (COPD) is pivotal for early diagnosis and management. While COPD develops gradually, early detection can significantly influence the course of the disease, allowing for interventions that may slow progression and improve quality of life.

Common Symptoms

COPD symptoms often don't appear until significant lung damage has occurred, and they usually worsen over time, particularly if smoking exposure continues. Key symptoms include:

- **Persistent Cough:** A cough that lingers for a long time, often termed as a smoker's cough, is one of the earliest signs of COPD.

- **Increased Mucus Production:** The production of a large amount of mucus or phlegm, especially in the morning, is common.

- **Breathlessness:** Initially, shortness of breath might only be noticeable during physical exertion. As the disease progresses, it can become a persistent issue, even during rest.

- **Wheezing:** A whistling or rattling sound when breathing, particularly during exhalation, indicates airflow obstruction.

- **Frequent Respiratory Infections:** Individuals with COPD may experience an increased frequency of colds, flu, or other respiratory infections.

Less Common Symptoms

In addition to the primary symptoms, there are several other signs that may indicate the presence of COPD or its complications, including:

- **Fatigue:** Chronic tiredness and lack of energy can be prominent as the disease advances, affecting daily activities and quality of life.

- **Weight Loss:** Advanced COPD can lead to weight loss and muscle wasting, partly due to the increased energy required for breathing and partly due to reduced food intake associated with breathlessness and fatigue.

- **Chest Tightness:** A sensation of tightness or discomfort in the chest is often reported, especially during episodes of increased breathlessness.

- **Cyanosis:** A bluish tint to the lips or fingernail beds (cyanosis) may occur due to low levels of oxygen in the blood.

When to Seek Medical Advice

It's crucial to seek medical advice if you or someone you know is experiencing these symptoms, especially if there's a history of risk factor exposure such as smoking or occupational hazards. Early consultation can lead to early diagnosis and management, significantly affecting the disease's trajectory.

Importance of Symptom Recognition

Recognizing the signs and symptoms of COPD is the first step in the journey toward management. It allows individuals and healthcare professionals to initiate conversations about lifestyle changes, particularly smoking cessation, and to explore diagnostic tests such as spirometry. Awareness and understanding of these symptoms foster a proactive approach to health, encouraging individuals to seek the necessary support and treatment to manage their condition effectively.

1.3 Risk Factors and Causes: A Deeper Dive

Understanding the risk factors and causes of Chronic Obstructive Pulmonary Disease (COPD) is crucial for prevention and early intervention. COPD is not caused by a single factor but rather a combination of environmental exposures and genetic predispositions that lead to the development of the disease. This section explores these risk factors in depth, offering insights into how each contributes to the onset and progression of COPD.

Tobacco Smoke

The primary and most significant risk factor for COPD is long-term exposure to tobacco smoke. This includes not only active smoking but also secondhand smoke exposure. The harmful chemicals in smoke can damage the lungs' airways and air sacs, leading to COPD in smokers and nonsmokers alike. The risk increases with the number and duration of years of smoking, making smoking cessation the most effective measure for preventing COPD.

Occupational Exposures

Exposure to dusts, chemicals, and fumes in the workplace can also significantly increase the risk of developing COPD. Occupations such as mining, welding, and construction, where workers are exposed to silica dust, asbestos, and other harmful substances, are particularly at risk. Protective measures and regulations to reduce exposure to these irritants can help lower the risk.

Air Pollution

Both indoor and outdoor air pollution are important risk factors for COPD. Inhaling polluted air, which contains particulate matter, ozone, nitrogen dioxide, and sulfur dioxide, can irritate the airways and lead to chronic respiratory conditions. Indoor air pollution, particularly from the use of biomass fuels (such as wood or coal) for cooking and heating in poorly ventilated spaces, is a significant risk factor in many parts of the world.

Genetic Factors

While less common, genetic predispositions can play a role in the development of COPD. The best-known genetic risk factor is a deficiency in alpha-1 antitrypsin (AAT), a protein that protects the lungs. Individuals with AAT deficiency are at a higher risk of developing COPD, especially if they smoke.

Age and Gender

The risk of developing COPD increases with age, as the cumulative exposure to risk factors tends to increase over time. Historically, COPD has been more prevalent in men, but the incidence in women is rising, likely due to increased tobacco use among women in recent decades.

Respiratory Infections

Frequent and severe respiratory infections during childhood and adulthood can contribute to the development of COPD by damaging the lung tissue. Ensuring good infection control and vaccination can help minimize this risk.

Socioeconomic Status

Socioeconomic factors play a significant role in the risk of developing COPD. Individuals from lower socioeconomic backgrounds are more likely to be exposed to the risk factors mentioned above, including tobacco smoke, occupational hazards, and indoor air pollution, due to living and working conditions.

Understanding and Mitigating Risk

Recognizing these risk factors is the first step in mitigating the risk of developing COPD. Lifestyle changes, particularly quitting smoking, reducing exposure to lung irritants, and improving living conditions, can significantly decrease the risk of COPD. Public health policies and individual actions aimed at addressing these risk factors are crucial for preventing the onset and progression of COPD.

1.4 Exercise: 10 MCQs with Answers at the End

Test your understanding of COPD with these multiple-choice questions. Answers are provided at the end for self-assessment.

1. What is the primary cause of COPD?

   A. Air pollution

   B. Genetic factors

   C. Tobacco smoke

   D. Respiratory infections

2. Which of the following is NOT a common symptom of COPD?

   A. Persistent cough

   B. Frequent nosebleeds

   C. Breathlessness

   D. Increased mucus production

3. COPD is characterized by which two main conditions?

   A. Asthma and pneumonia

   B. Emphysema and chronic bronchitis

   C. Tuberculosis and lung cancer

D. Cystic fibrosis and pulmonary fibrosis

4. How is COPD primarily diagnosed?

A. Chest X-Ray

B. Spirometry test

C. Complete blood count (CBC)

D. MRI of the chest

5. Which occupational exposure can increase the risk of developing COPD?

A. Prolonged sitting

B. Exposure to loud noises

C. Inhalation of chemical fumes

D. Frequent use of computer screens

6. What role does alpha-1 antitrypsin (AAT) play in COPD?

A. It causes the airways to constrict.

B. It protects the lungs from damage.

C. It increases mucus production.

D. It decreases oxygen uptake.

7. Which lifestyle change is most effective in preventing COPD?

A. Increased physical activity

B. Smoking cessation

C. High protein diet

D. Regular use of air purifiers

8. What is a significant risk factor for COPD not related to lifestyle or genetics?

A. High blood pressure

B. Air pollution

C. Excessive alcohol consumption

D. High cholesterol levels

9. Indoor air pollution is a risk factor for COPD. Which of the following contributes to indoor air pollution?

A. Use of biomass fuels for cooking and heating

B. Electric heating systems

C. Use of LED lighting

D. High-efficiency particulate air (HEPA) filters

10. Why are frequent and severe respiratory infections considered a risk factor for COPD?

A. They can cause genetic mutations leading to COPD.

B. They increase the risk of heart disease, which is related to COPD.

C. They can damage lung tissue and exacerbate the progression of COPD.

D. They lead to temporary lung function impairment, misdiagnosed as COPD.

Answers:

1. C. Tobacco smoke

2. B. Frequent nosebleeds

3. B. Emphysema and chronic bronchitis

4. B. Spirometry test

5. C. Inhalation of chemical fumes

6. B. It protects the lungs from damage.

7. B. Smoking cessation

8. B. Air pollution

9. A. Use of biomass fuels for cooking and heating

10. C. They can damage lung tissue and exacerbate the progression of COPD.

Chapter 2: Diagnosing COPD

2.1 The Role of Spirometry

Spirometry: The Diagnostic Cornerstone

Spirometry is the most important and widely used diagnostic test for Chronic Obstructive Pulmonary Disease (COPD). It measures the amount (volume) and/or speed (flow) of air that can be inhaled and exhaled, providing a clear picture of lung function and helping to identify the presence of obstruction or restriction in the airways.

How Spirometry Works

The test is simple, non-invasive, and involves blowing as hard as possible into a small, handheld device called a spirometer. The key measurements taken during the test include:

- **Forced Vital Capacity (FVC):** The maximum amount of air a person can exhale forcefully after a deep breath.

- **Forced Expiratory Volume in 1 Second (FEV1):** The amount of air a person can forcefully exhale in one second.

The FEV1/FVC ratio is then calculated to determine the presence of airflow obstruction, a hallmark of COPD. In individuals with COPD, this ratio is significantly lower than normal due to the difficulty in expelling air from the lungs.

Interpreting Spirometry Results

Spirometry results are interpreted based on reference values that consider age, sex, height, and ethnicity. A diagnosis of COPD is considered when the FEV1/FVC ratio is less than 70% after the administration of a bronchodilator, which helps to rule out asthma by reversing any reversible airflow obstruction.

The Importance of Spirometry in COPD Diagnosis

Early diagnosis of COPD through spirometry allows for prompt management and treatment, potentially slowing the progression of the disease. It is also useful in differentiating COPD from other respiratory conditions like asthma, which have different treatment protocols.

Spirometry in COPD Management

Beyond diagnosis, spirometry is essential in the ongoing management of COPD. It helps in assessing the severity of the disease, monitoring disease progression, and evaluating the effectiveness of prescribed treatments. Regular spirometry tests can guide adjustments in therapy to better control symptoms and improve quality of life.

Limitations and Considerations

While spirometry is invaluable in diagnosing and managing COPD, it is not without limitations. Accurate results depend on the patient's effort and cooperation, as well as the proper functioning and calibration of the spirometer. Additionally, spirometry cannot provide information about the underlying cause of the obstruction. Therefore, it is often used in conjunction with other tests and assessments to get a comprehensive understanding of a patient's respiratory health.

Conclusion

The role of spirometry in diagnosing and managing COPD cannot be overstated. It is a critical tool that provides objective data about lung function, aiding in the accurate diagnosis of COPD, distinguishing it from other respiratory conditions, and guiding effective treatment strategies. By embracing spirometry, healthcare providers can offer timely interventions, ultimately improving outcomes for individuals with COPD.

2.2 Other Diagnostic Tests and Procedures

While spirometry is the cornerstone of diagnosing Chronic Obstructive Pulmonary Disease (COPD), several other diagnostic tests and procedures are vital for a comprehensive assessment of the condition. These tests help to determine the severity of the disease, identify any complications, and plan the most effective treatment strategy.

Chest X-Ray

A chest X-ray is often one of the first tests performed in the evaluation of COPD. It can show signs of lung hyperinflation, flattened diaphragm curves indicative of emphysema, or reveal other conditions that might mimic or complicate COPD, such as pneumonia or heart failure.

CT Scan

A high-resolution computed tomography (CT) scan of the chest provides detailed images of the lungs and airways. It is particularly useful in detecting the presence and extent of emphysema, assessing chronic bronchitis, and identifying any structural abnormalities of the lungs. CT scans can also help in planning for certain surgical treatments.

Arterial Blood Gas Analysis

This test measures the levels of oxygen and carbon dioxide in the arterial blood. It helps assess the severity of COPD and whether oxygen therapy might be needed. A low level of oxygen (hypoxemia) and a high level of carbon dioxide (hypercapnia) in the blood can indicate advanced COPD.

Pulmonary Function Tests (PFTs)

Besides spirometry, other pulmonary function tests may be performed to get a more complete picture of lung function. These include measurements of lung volumes, diffusion capacity (DLCO), which assesses how well gases are transferred from the lungs to the blood, and respiratory muscle strength tests.

Alpha-1 Antitrypsin Deficiency Screening

Since alpha-1 antitrypsin deficiency is a genetic risk factor for COPD, particularly emphysema, screening for this condition is recommended for individuals with COPD, especially if they have a family history of the disease or develop COPD at a young age or without a history of smoking.

Oximetry

Pulse oximetry is a non-invasive test that measures the oxygen saturation level of the blood. It's a simple, quick test that can be used to monitor the severity of COPD and the effectiveness of oxygen therapy.

Exercise Testing

Exercise tests, such as the six-minute walk test (6MWT), can evaluate the functional status of individuals with COPD. These tests measure the distance walked on a flat, hard surface in a specified period, indicating the person's exercise capacity and endurance.

Sputum Examination

Analysis of sputum can help identify infections or the presence of inflammatory cells, which can guide the choice of antibiotics or corticosteroids in treating exacerbations of COPD.

Conclusion

The comprehensive evaluation of COPD often requires a combination of these diagnostic tests and procedures. Each provides unique information that contributes to a fuller understanding of the disease's impact on the individual. This holistic approach enables tailored treatment plans that address the specific needs and challenges faced by those living with COPD, optimizing outcomes and enhancing quality of life.

2.3 Interpreting Test Results

Interpreting the results of diagnostic tests for Chronic Obstructive Pulmonary Disease (COPD) is a critical step in confirming the diagnosis, assessing the severity of the disease, and guiding treatment decisions. This section provides an overview of how healthcare providers interpret the results from various diagnostic tests and what these results indicate about a patient's lung health.

Spirometry

- **FEV1/FVC Ratio:** The ratio of Forced Expiratory Volume in 1 second (FEV1) to Forced Vital Capacity (FVC) is used to diagnose airflow obstruction. A ratio less than 0.70 (70%) post-bronchodilator administration confirms persistent airflow limitation, indicative of COPD.

- **FEV1:** The absolute value of FEV1, often expressed as a percentage of the predicted value based on the patient's age, sex, height, and ethnicity, is used to gauge the severity of airflow obstruction.

Staging of COPD Severity (GOLD Guidelines):

- **Mild (GOLD 1):** FEV1 ≥ 80% predicted

- **Moderate (GOLD 2):** 50% ≤ FEV1 < 80% predicted

- **Severe (GOLD 3):** 30% ≤ FEV1 < 50% predicted

- **Very Severe (GOLD 4):** FEV1 < 30% predicted

Chest X-Ray and CT Scan

- **Emphysema:** Visible as areas of decreased lung density, enlarged air spaces, and a reduced vascular pattern.

- **Chronic Bronchitis:** May show increased lung markings and evidence of bronchial wall thickening.

- **Signs of Complications:** Such as pneumonia or pneumothorax, are also assessed.

Arterial Blood Gas Analysis

- **Hypoxemia:** A reduced level of oxygen in the blood, indicating impaired gas exchange.

- **Hypercapnia:** An increased level of carbon dioxide in the blood, suggesting advanced disease with poor ventilation.

Pulmonary Function Tests (PFTs)

- **Lung Volumes and Capacities:** Increased residual volume (RV) and total lung capacity (TLC) can indicate hyperinflation due to air trapping.

- **Diffusion Capacity (DLCO):** Decreased DLCO suggests impaired gas exchange across the alveolar-capillary membrane, common in emphysema.

Alpha-1 Antitrypsin Deficiency Screening

- A significantly low level of alpha-1 antitrypsin suggests a genetic predisposition to developing COPD, particularly emphysema, even in non-smokers.

Oximetry and Exercise Testing

- **Decreased Oxygen Saturation:** Indicates the need for supplemental oxygen.

- **Exercise Capacity:** Reduced exercise tolerance as evidenced by tests like the 6-minute walk test can help in assessing disease impact and guiding rehabilitation efforts.

Sputum Examination

- **Infectious Agents:** Identification of bacteria or viruses can guide antibiotic or antiviral therapy.

- **Inflammatory Cells:** Presence of eosinophils or neutrophils can indicate the type of inflammation and guide steroid use.

Interpreting Test Results in Context

Interpreting these test results requires consideration of the complete clinical picture, including symptoms, physical examination findings, and patient history. For example, a patient with a FEV1/FVC ratio of less than 0.70 and symptoms of chronic cough and breathlessness likely has COPD, but the severity and specific treatment approach depend on additional factors like symptom burden, exacerbation history, and comorbid conditions.

Dynamic Nature of COPD

It's also important to recognize that COPD is a dynamic disease. Regular monitoring and reassessment using these tests are essential for adjusting treatment plans as the disease progresses or improves with treatment. This holistic and dynamic approach to interpreting test results is crucial for providing personalized care to individuals with COPD, ensuring that management strategies are tailored to their evolving needs.

2.4 Exercise: 10 MCQs with Answers at the End

Test your knowledge on diagnosing COPD with these multiple-choice questions. Answers are provided at the end for self-assessment.

1. What is the primary function of spirometry in diagnosing COPD?

   A. To measure lung volumes

   B. To assess the diffusion capacity

   C. To identify the presence of airflow obstruction

   D. To check for respiratory infections

2. What does a FEV1/FVC ratio less than 0.70 indicate?

   A. Asthma

   B. COPD

   C. Pulmonary fibrosis

   D. Healthy lung function

3. Which imaging test is commonly used to identify emphysema in COPD patients?

A. MRI

B. CT scan

C. Chest X-Ray

D. Ultrasound

4. What does arterial blood gas analysis primarily assess in COPD patients?

A. Nutrient levels

B. Infection presence

C. Gas exchange efficiency

D. Blood pH level

5. The GOLD guidelines classify COPD severity based on which spirometry result?

A. Total Lung Capacity (TLC)

B. Forced Expiratory Volume in 1 second (FEV1)

C. Peak Expiratory Flow (PEF)

D. Forced Vital Capacity (FVC)

6. A high-resolution CT scan in COPD can show all of the following EXCEPT:

A. Air trapping

B. Pulmonary hypertension

C. Bronchial wall thickening

D. Enlarged air spaces

7. Which test is used for genetic screening for COPD risk?

A. Complete blood count (CBC)

B. Alpha-1 antitrypsin deficiency screening

C. Lipid profile

D. Electrolyte panel

8. Pulse oximetry measures:

A. Carbon dioxide levels in blood

B. Oxygen saturation levels in blood

C. Blood pressure

D. Heart rate

9. The six-minute walk test (6MWT) is used to assess:

A. Cognitive function

B. Exercise capacity

C. Lung function

D. Cardiac function

10. A decreased diffusion capacity (DLCO) suggests:

A. Impaired gas exchange across the lung membrane

B. Increased risk of lung infections

C. High blood oxygen levels

D. Efficient removal of carbon dioxide from the blood

Answers:

1. C. To identify the presence of airflow obstruction

2. B. COPD

3. B. CT scan

4. C. Gas exchange efficiency

5. B. Forced Expiratory Volume in 1 second (FEV1)

6. B. Pulmonary hypertension

7. B. Alpha-1 antitrypsin deficiency screening

8. B. Oxygen saturation levels in blood

9. B. Exercise capacity

10. A. Impaired gas exchange across the lung membrane

Chapter 3: The Impact of COPD on Daily Life

3.1 Physical Limitations and Adaptations

Understanding the Physical Impact

Chronic Obstructive Pulmonary Disease (COPD) significantly affects the physical capabilities of those diagnosed with the condition. The progressive nature of COPD means that physical limitations often increase over time, impacting daily activities, mobility, and overall quality of life. Understanding these limitations is crucial for managing COPD effectively and making necessary adaptations to maintain as much independence and activity as possible.

Common Physical Limitations

- **Breathlessness:** Shortness of breath, especially during physical activities, is a hallmark symptom of COPD. This can make routine tasks such as walking, climbing stairs, or even dressing, challenging.

- **Fatigue:** People with COPD often experience increased fatigue, not just because of the extra effort needed to breathe but also due to disrupted sleep patterns and the body's effort to compensate for decreased oxygen levels.

- **Exercise Intolerance:** Reduced exercise capacity is common, making it hard to engage in physical activities that were once easy or enjoyable. This can lead to a decrease in physical fitness, further exacerbating symptoms.

- **Muscle Weakness:** Decreased muscle mass and strength, particularly in the legs, can occur due to reduced activity levels and systemic effects of COPD.

Adaptations for Managing Physical Limitations

Adapting to these physical limitations requires a comprehensive approach, involving lifestyle changes, pulmonary rehabilitation, and modifications to the living environment.

- **Pulmonary Rehabilitation:** This program combines exercise training, education, and support to help people with COPD improve their physical and emotional well-being. It teaches patients how to exercise safely and effectively, manage breathlessness, and conserve energy.

- **Energy Conservation Techniques:** Simple strategies can make daily tasks less taxing. Planning and pacing activities, sitting for tasks that can be done seated, and using labor-saving devices can help conserve energy.

- **Exercise and Physical Activity:** Tailored exercise programs can help improve exercise tolerance, muscle strength, and overall fitness. Activities like walking, cycling, and strength training, adjusted to individual capabilities, can have significant benefits.

- **Home Modifications:** Making changes to the living environment can help minimize the impact of physical limitations. This might include installing grab bars in the bathroom, using a shower chair, or keeping everyday items within easy reach to reduce the need for bending or stretching.

Emotional and Social Support

In addition to these physical adaptations, emotional and social support is vital. Coping with the physical limitations of COPD can be challenging, and support from family, friends, and support groups can provide encouragement, practical advice, and a sense of community.

Conclusion

Living with COPD requires adjustments to manage the physical limitations imposed by the disease. Through pulmonary rehabilitation, energy conservation techniques, tailored exercise, and home modifications, individuals with COPD can maintain a level of independence and quality of life. Recognizing these limitations and making appropriate adaptations is a key step in managing COPD effectively.

3.2 Emotional and Psychological Considerations

Navigating Emotional and Psychological Challenges

Chronic Obstructive Pulmonary Disease (COPD) not only imposes physical limitations but also brings significant emotional and psychological challenges. The chronic nature of the disease, coupled with its impact on daily life and independence, can lead to a range of emotional responses, including anxiety, depression, and fear. Addressing these aspects is crucial for comprehensive COPD management and improving overall well-being.

Common Emotional Responses

- **Anxiety and Panic:** Breathlessness, a core symptom of COPD, can trigger anxiety and panic attacks, creating a vicious cycle that can exacerbate symptoms.

- **Depression:** The ongoing struggles and limitations imposed by COPD can lead to feelings of sadness, hopelessness, and depression, affecting the motivation to engage in treatment and self-care.

- **Fear of Progression:** Many individuals experience fear regarding the progression of their disease and the potential for future exacerbations, impacting their quality of life and emotional well-being.

- **Social Isolation:** Physical limitations and the effort required to manage COPD symptoms can lead to withdrawal from social activities, increasing feelings of isolation and loneliness.

Strategies for Managing Emotional and Psychological Impact

- **Pulmonary Rehabilitation:** Beyond physical benefits, pulmonary rehabilitation offers psychological support, helping individuals understand their condition, manage symptoms, and address fears and anxieties.

- **Counseling and Support Groups:** Professional counseling and participation in COPD support groups can provide a valuable outlet for sharing experiences and coping strategies, reducing feelings of isolation.

- **Stress Management Techniques:** Techniques such as deep breathing, mindfulness, and meditation can help manage anxiety and stress, improving emotional regulation and reducing panic attacks related to breathlessness.

- **Regular Exercise:** Physical activity can enhance mood and reduce symptoms of depression and anxiety, contributing to overall emotional well-being.

- **Education and Self-Management:** Understanding COPD and learning how to manage it can empower individuals, reduce fear of the unknown, and help regain a sense of control over their lives.

The Role of Healthcare Providers

Healthcare providers play a critical role in recognizing the emotional and psychological needs of individuals with COPD. Regular screening for symptoms of anxiety and depression, providing information on available resources, and referrals to mental health professionals when necessary are essential components of comprehensive COPD care.

Conclusion

The emotional and psychological considerations of living with COPD are as significant as the physical aspects of the disease. Addressing these concerns through comprehensive care that includes psychological support, education, and strategies for managing stress and emotions is vital. By acknowledging and tackling these challenges, individuals with COPD can improve their quality of life, enhance their ability to manage the disease, and foster a more positive outlook on living with COPD.

3.3 Social and Family Dynamics

Living with Chronic Obstructive Pulmonary Disease (COPD) affects not just the individual diagnosed but also their social and family dynamics. The disease can significantly alter relationships, roles within the family, and social interactions, requiring adjustments from both the person with COPD and their loved ones.

Impact on Family Roles and Relationships

- **Caregiving Responsibilities:** Family members often become caregivers, a role that can be both rewarding and challenging, potentially leading to stress and caregiver burnout.

- **Changed Family Dynamics:** As the person with COPD may no longer be able to fulfill certain roles or tasks they previously managed, this shift can affect family dynamics and responsibilities, requiring adaptation and negotiation.

- **Emotional Strain:** The emotional and psychological impact of COPD on the patient can also affect family members, who may experience feelings of worry, sadness, or frustration.

Maintaining Social Connections

COPD can lead to a decrease in social activities due to physical limitations, fatigue, and the need for frequent rest. This reduction in social engagement can contribute to feelings of isolation and loneliness, not only for the individual with COPD but also for their caregivers.

Strategies for Supporting Social and Family Dynamics

- **Open Communication:** Encouraging open and honest communication within the family and with friends about the challenges and needs associated with COPD can foster understanding and support.

- **Seeking Support:** Utilizing support groups and counseling services can provide emotional support and practical advice for both individuals with COPD and their family members.

- **Setting Realistic Expectations:** Adjusting expectations regarding activities, responsibilities, and social engagements can help in managing the impact of COPD on daily life.

- **Shared Decision Making:** Involving all family members in care planning and decision-making can promote a sense of teamwork and shared responsibility, easing the burden on any one individual.

- **Educating Family and Friends:** Providing education about COPD to family and friends can help them understand the condition, its effects, and how they can offer effective support.

Conclusion

The influence of COPD on social and family dynamics underscores the importance of addressing not just the physical aspects of the disease but also its broader implications. By fostering open communication, seeking support, and adjusting expectations, families can navigate the challenges of COPD together, strengthening their relationships and improving the quality of life for everyone involved. This holistic approach to COPD care ensures that both individuals with COPD and their loved ones are supported throughout the journey.

3.4 Exercise: 10 MCQs with Answers at the End

Evaluate your understanding of the impact of COPD on daily life, including physical, emotional, social, and family dynamics, with these multiple-choice questions. Answers are provided at the end for self-assessment.

1. What is a common physical limitation experienced by individuals with COPD?

   A. Increased muscle strength

   B. Breathlessness

   C. Improved exercise tolerance

   D. Decreased fatigue

2. Pulmonary rehabilitation programs for COPD patients primarily aim to:

   A. Cure COPD

   B. Improve emotional well-being only

   C. Improve physical and emotional well-being

   D. Increase lung capacity

3. Which of the following is NOT a common emotional response to COPD?

A. Joy

B. Anxiety

C. Depression

D. Fear of progression

4. Stress management techniques beneficial for COPD patients include:

A. Avoiding all physical activity

B. Deep breathing exercises

C. Increasing smoking

D. Limiting social interactions

5. The role of caregivers in managing COPD may lead to:

A. Decreased stress

B. Caregiver burnout

C. Less responsibility

D. Improved personal health

6. Maintaining social connections with COPD can be challenging due to:

A. Enhanced mobility

B. Increased energy levels

C. Physical limitations and fatigue

D. Decreased need for rest

7. Open communication within the family about COPD can:

A. Increase misunderstandings

B. Foster understanding and support

C. Lead to isolation

D. Reduce the need for medical care

8. Shared decision making in COPD care encourages:

A. Dependence on one family member

B. A sense of teamwork and shared responsibility

C. Ignoring the patient's preferences

D. Decreased family involvement

9. Education about COPD for family and friends is important because it:

A. Decreases their willingness to help

B. Increases anxiety and worry

C. Helps them understand the condition and how to offer support

D. Is unnecessary if the patient understands their condition

10. Effective support for a loved one with COPD includes:

A. Encouraging physical and social activity within their limits

B. Telling them to manage on their own to increase independence

C. Avoiding discussions about the disease

D. Insisting on doing everything for them to reduce their burden

Answers:

1. B. Breathlessness

2. C. Improve physical and emotional well-being

3. A. Joy

4. B. Deep breathing exercises

5. B. Caregiver burnout

6. C. Physical limitations and fatigue

7. B. Foster understanding and support

8. B. A sense of teamwork and shared responsibility

9. C. Helps them understand the condition and how to offer support

10. A. Encouraging physical and social activity within their limits

Chapter 4: Treatment Strategies for COPD

4.1 Medications and Therapies

Overview

While there is no cure for Chronic Obstructive Pulmonary Disease (COPD), a range of medications and therapies are available that can help control symptoms, reduce the frequency and severity of exacerbations, and improve quality of life. Treatment plans are tailored to the individual's symptoms, disease severity, and overall health status.

Bronchodilators

Bronchodilators are the cornerstone of COPD treatment. They work by relaxing the muscles around the airways, making it easier to breathe. There are two main types:

- **Short-acting bronchodilators** provide quick relief from symptoms and are often used on an "as-needed" basis.

- **Long-acting bronchodilators** are used daily to provide ongoing symptom control and improve lung function.

Bronchodilators are available in two classes: beta2-agonists and anticholinergics, and they may be used alone or in combination.

Inhaled Corticosteroids (ICS)

For individuals with frequent exacerbations or more severe disease, inhaled corticosteroids can be added to reduce inflammation in the airways, improve symptoms, and decrease the frequency of flare-ups. However, they are not recommended for long-term use in all COPD patients due to potential side effects.

Combination Inhalers

Combination inhalers that include both a bronchodilator and a corticosteroid can simplify the treatment regimen and improve adherence. There are also inhalers that combine two different classes of bronchodilators for even better control of symptoms.

Phosphodiesterase-4 Inhibitors

This class of medication targets inflammation and is specifically designed for individuals with chronic bronchitis and a history of exacerbations. It is usually prescribed when symptoms are not adequately controlled by bronchodilators alone.

Oxygen Therapy

For patients with severe COPD and low oxygen levels, long-term oxygen therapy can improve survival, ease symptoms, increase exercise tolerance, and improve quality of life.

Pulmonary Rehabilitation

Pulmonary rehabilitation is a comprehensive program that combines exercise, education, and support to help people with COPD improve their physical and psychological condition. It is tailored to the individual's needs and can help reduce breathlessness, increase exercise capacity, and improve the overall quality of life.

Vaccinations

Annual flu vaccines and pneumococcal vaccines are recommended for all individuals with COPD to reduce the risk of respiratory infections, which can trigger exacerbations.

Antibiotics

Antibiotics may be prescribed during exacerbations if there is evidence of bacterial infection. Some patients with frequent exacerbations might be given antibiotics to take at the first sign of an infection as part of a self-management plan.

Conclusion

Managing COPD requires a multifaceted approach that includes medications, therapies, and lifestyle modifications. Regular follow-up with healthcare providers is essential to monitor disease progression, adjust treatment plans as needed, and address any new symptoms or concerns. With effective management, individuals with COPD can achieve better control of their symptoms, reduce the risk of exacerbations, and maintain an active and fulfilling life.

4.2 Pulmonary Rehabilitation: Techniques and Benefits

Pulmonary Rehabilitation Overview

Pulmonary rehabilitation (PR) is a comprehensive intervention designed for patients with chronic respiratory diseases, including COPD. It combines various techniques to improve the physical and psychological condition of patients, aiming to enhance the overall quality of life. PR is highly individualized, taking into account the specific needs, abilities, and objectives of each patient.

Core Components of Pulmonary Rehabilitation

- **Exercise Training:** Tailored exercise programs focus on improving cardiovascular fitness, muscle strength, and endurance. Aerobic exercises (like walking or cycling) and strength training are central, helping to reduce breathlessness and fatigue.

- **Education:** Patients receive education on COPD management, including understanding the disease, medication usage, nutritional advice, and strategies to conserve energy and manage breathlessness.

- **Breathing Techniques:** Techniques such as pursed-lip breathing and diaphragmatic breathing are taught to help control breathlessness during activities.

- **Psychological Support:** Counseling and support groups are offered to address the emotional aspects of living with COPD, including coping strategies for anxiety and depression.

Benefits of Pulmonary Rehabilitation

- **Improved Exercise Tolerance:** One of the most significant benefits is increased exercise capacity, which translates to better endurance for daily activities.

- **Symptom Management:** PR helps to reduce symptoms of breathlessness and fatigue, making it easier for patients to engage in physical activities and maintain independence.

- **Enhanced Quality of Life:** By addressing physical and psychological needs, PR significantly improves the overall quality of life for patients with COPD.

- **Reduced Hospitalizations:** Participation in a PR program can lead to fewer exacerbations and hospital admissions.

- **Increased Knowledge:** Patients gain a better understanding of their condition, which empowers them to take an active role in managing their health.

- **Social Support:** Group sessions provide a sense of community, reducing feelings of isolation by connecting patients with others who are facing similar challenges.

Who Can Benefit?

Pulmonary rehabilitation is beneficial at all stages of COPD, from mild to very severe. Candidates include individuals who experience breathlessness or other respiratory symptoms that interfere with their daily activities, regardless of their lung function test results.

Conclusion

Pulmonary rehabilitation is a cornerstone in the management of COPD, offering a holistic approach to care that addresses the physical, emotional, and social impacts of the disease. Through a combination of exercise, education, and support, PR empowers patients to improve their health and quality of life, despite the challenges of living with a chronic respiratory condition. Regular participation and adherence to the principles learned in PR can lead to sustained benefits and a more active, fulfilling life.

4.3 Surgical Options and Considerations

Introduction to Surgical Interventions for COPD

For certain individuals with Chronic Obstructive Pulmonary Disease (COPD), medical management and pulmonary rehabilitation may not sufficiently alleviate symptoms or improve quality of life. In these cases, surgical interventions may be considered as part of a comprehensive treatment plan. Surgical options are generally reserved for patients with specific disease characteristics and those who have not responded adequately to other treatments.

Types of Surgical Interventions

- **Lung Volume Reduction Surgery (LVRS):** LVRS involves the removal of diseased, emphysematous lung tissue, which can improve lung function, decrease breathlessness, and enhance the patient's ability to exercise. This surgery is typically considered for patients with severe emphysema who have excessive lung volume.

- **Bullectomy:** A bullectomy is the surgical removal of a bulla, a large air space within the lung that can compress healthy lung tissue. Removing the bulla can help improve lung function and alleviate symptoms in patients with large bullae.

- **Lung Transplantation:** In advanced cases of COPD, a lung transplant may be considered. This involves replacing the diseased lung(s) with a healthy lung(s) from a donor. Lung transplantation is a complex procedure with significant risks and requires a lifelong commitment to medication and care to prevent organ rejection.

Considerations Before Surgery

- **Patient Selection:** Not all patients with COPD are candidates for surgery. Factors such as the patient's overall health, lung function, disease distribution within the lungs, and smoking status are critical in determining eligibility.

- **Risks and Benefits:** Surgical options carry risks, including complications from the surgery itself and the potential for postoperative infections. The expected benefits, such as improved lung function and quality of life, must outweigh these risks for surgery to be considered.

- **Postoperative Care:** Successful surgery requires a commitment to postoperative care, including participation in pulmonary rehabilitation, adherence to medication, and lifestyle changes, such as smoking cessation.

- **Multidisciplinary Evaluation:** A thorough evaluation by a multidisciplinary team, including pulmonologists, thoracic surgeons, and other specialists, is essential to assess suitability for surgery and to plan the best approach.

Outcomes and Quality of Life

Surgical interventions can offer significant improvements in symptoms, exercise tolerance, and quality of life for selected patients with COPD. However, these benefits must be balanced against the potential risks and the need for comprehensive postoperative care.

Conclusion

Surgical options for COPD, such as LVRS, bullectomy, and lung transplantation, can be life-changing for patients who are appropriate candidates. These interventions are considered within the broader context of the patient's COPD management plan, emphasizing the importance of careful patient selection, detailed preoperative assessment, and dedicated postoperative care to optimize outcomes.

4.4 Exercise: 10 MCQs with Answers at the End

Evaluate your knowledge on the treatment strategies for COPD, including medications, therapies, surgical options, and their considerations, with these multiple-choice questions. Answers are provided at the end for self-assessment.

1. What is the primary goal of bronchodilators in COPD treatment?

   A. Cure COPD

   B. Suppress the immune system

   C. Relieve breathlessness and improve airflow

   D. Increase oxygen levels in the blood

2. Inhaled corticosteroids (ICS) are primarily prescribed for COPD patients with:

   A. Mild symptoms and no history of exacerbations

   B. Frequent exacerbations

   C. High blood pressure

   D. Allergy to beta2-agonists

3. Which type of medication is specifically designed to target inflammation in patients with chronic bronchitis and a history of exacerbations?

A. Beta2-agonists

B. Phosphodiesterase-4 inhibitors

C. Anticholinergics

D. Antibiotics

4. The main focus of pulmonary rehabilitation is to:

A. Perform surgery on the lungs

B. Improve physical and emotional well-being

C. Increase lung volume

D. Provide oxygen therapy

5. Lung Volume Reduction Surgery (LVRS) is most beneficial for patients with:

A. Mild COPD

B. Severe emphysema and excessive lung volume

C. Early-stage chronic bronchitis

D. COPD without emphysema

6. The purpose of a bullectomy is to:

   A. Remove a portion of the lung's airways

   B. Replace the diseased lung with a healthy one

   C. Remove large air spaces (bullae) from the lungs

   D. Increase blood flow to the lungs

7. Lung transplantation in COPD patients is:

   A. A first-line treatment option

   B. Recommended for all patients with severe COPD

   C. Considered for advanced cases when other treatments have failed

   D. Only performed in patients younger than 40 years old

8. Which statement about pulmonary rehabilitation is TRUE?

   A. It eliminates the need for medication in COPD

   B. Only focuses on physical exercises

   C. Offers psychological support and education

   D. Is a short-term solution with temporary benefits

9. Annual vaccinations recommended for COPD patients include:

   A. Hepatitis B vaccine

   B. Flu vaccine and pneumococcal vaccine

   C. Human papillomavirus (HPV) vaccine

D. Measles, mumps, and rubella (MMR) vaccine

10. The multidisciplinary evaluation for surgical options in COPD does NOT include:

A. Pulmonologists

B. Thoracic surgeons

C. Nutritionists only

D. Other specialists like cardiologists

Answers:

1. C. Relieve breathlessness and improve airflow

2. B. Frequent exacerbations

3. B. Phosphodiesterase-4 inhibitors

4. B. Improve physical and emotional well-being

5. B. Severe emphysema and excessive lung volume

6. C. Remove large air spaces (bullae) from the lungs

7. C. Considered for advanced cases when other treatments have failed

8. C. Offers psychological support and education

9. B. Flu vaccine and pneumococcal vaccine

10. C. Nutritionists only

Chapter 5: Lifestyle Modifications and COPD Management

5.1 Diet and Nutrition: Fueling Your Lungs

The Role of Diet in COPD Management

Proper nutrition plays a crucial role in managing Chronic Obstructive Pulmonary Disease (COPD). A balanced diet can help maintain an optimal body weight, improve lung function, and enhance the body's ability to fight infections. Nutritional advice for COPD patients often focuses on preventing malnutrition, managing symptoms, and supporting overall health.

Nutritional Challenges in COPD

COPD patients may face unique nutritional challenges, including:

- **Weight Loss and Muscle Wasting:** Increased energy expenditure due to the effort of breathing and systemic inflammation can lead to unintentional weight loss and muscle wasting.

- **Overweight and Obesity:** Conversely, some individuals may struggle with being overweight, which can exacerbate breathing difficulties.

- **Difficulty Eating:** Breathlessness and fatigue can make the physical act of eating exhausting.

Key Dietary Recommendations

- **High-Protein Foods:** Protein is essential for maintaining muscle strength, including the respiratory muscles. Incorporate lean meats, fish, eggs, dairy, and legumes into your diet.

- **Energy-Dense Foods:** For those struggling with weight loss, energy-dense foods can help meet calorie needs without requiring large volumes of food. Nuts, seeds, and avocados are good options.

- **Fruits and Vegetables:** Rich in vitamins, minerals, and antioxidants, fruits and vegetables can help combat inflammation and support immune function.

- **Whole Grains:** Provide essential nutrients and fiber, which can help maintain a healthy digestive system.

- **Healthy Fats:** Omega-3 fatty acids found in fish oil, flaxseeds, and walnuts have anti-inflammatory properties, which can be beneficial for COPD patients.

- **Hydration:** Adequate fluid intake helps thin mucus, making it easier to clear from the lungs.

Managing Weight Issues

- **For Underweight Patients:** Focus on frequent, small, nutrient- and calorie-dense meals. Consider working with a dietitian to ensure you're getting enough calories and nutrients.

- **For Overweight Patients:** A balanced diet with controlled portion sizes and a focus on nutrient-dense foods can help achieve a healthier weight, reducing the strain on the respiratory system.

Special Considerations

- **Salt Intake:** Excessive salt can lead to fluid retention, worsening breathlessness. Aim for a low-sodium diet.

- **Dietary Supplements:** Some patients may benefit from dietary supplements, but it's important to consult with a healthcare provider before starting any new supplement, as some may interact with medications.

Conclusion

Diet and nutrition are integral components of COPD management, with the potential to significantly impact symptom control, disease progression, and overall quality of life. Tailoring dietary intake to meet the individual needs of COPD patients, considering their specific health status and nutritional challenges, can help optimize their respiratory function and enhance their well-being.

5.2 Exercise and Physical Activity

The Importance of Exercise in COPD Management

Exercise plays a critical role in managing Chronic Obstructive Pulmonary Disease (COPD). While it might seem counterintuitive for individuals who experience breathlessness to engage in physical activity, regular exercise can significantly improve lung function, increase stamina, reduce symptoms, and enhance overall quality of life.

Benefits of Regular Exercise for COPD Patients

- **Improved Cardiovascular Health:** Exercise strengthens the heart and improves circulation, helping to deliver oxygen more efficiently throughout the body.

- **Increased Muscle Strength:** Strengthening the muscles, especially those used for breathing, can ease the workload on the lungs.

- **Enhanced Endurance:** Regular physical activity improves stamina, making daily activities easier to perform.

- **Better Control of Symptoms:** Exercise can help reduce the severity of breathlessness and fatigue.

- **Improved Mental Health:** Regular exercise has been shown to reduce anxiety and depression, which are common among individuals with COPD.

Recommended Types of Exercise

- **Aerobic Exercise:** Activities like walking, cycling, and swimming increase heart rate and improve lung function. These exercises should be done at a moderate intensity, where conversation is possible but requires some effort.

- **Strength Training:** Working with weights or resistance bands strengthens the muscles, making everyday activities easier and improving metabolic rate.

- **Flexibility Exercises:** Stretching helps maintain mobility and reduce the risk of injury.

- **Breathing Exercises:** Techniques such as pursed-lip breathing and diaphragmatic breathing can help manage shortness of breath during physical activity.

Creating an Exercise Plan

It's important for COPD patients to work with their healthcare provider or a pulmonary rehabilitation specialist to develop an exercise plan tailored to their specific needs and abilities. Here are some tips for creating an effective exercise regimen:

- **Start Slowly:** Begin with short sessions of light activity and gradually increase duration and intensity based on tolerance and improvement in symptoms.

- **Incorporate Variety:** A mix of aerobic, strength, and flexibility exercises can provide comprehensive benefits.

- **Listen to Your Body:** Adjust the intensity of exercise based on how you feel. Utilize breathing techniques to manage shortness of breath.

- **Stay Consistent:** Regular exercise yields the best results. Aim for at least 30 minutes of moderate exercise most days of the week.

Safety Considerations

- **Monitor Symptoms:** Pay attention to signs of overexertion, such as increased breathlessness, chest pain, or dizziness.

- **Use Oxygen if Prescribed:** Those on supplemental oxygen should use it during exercise as directed by their healthcare provider.

- **Stay Hydrated:** Proper hydration is essential, especially during physical activity.

Conclusion

Exercise is a cornerstone of effective COPD management, offering numerous benefits that extend beyond lung function to impact overall health and well-being. With careful planning, regular monitoring, and appropriate adjustments, physical activity can be a safe and effective way for individuals with COPD to improve their quality of life.

5.3 Quitting Smoking: Tips and Strategies

The Impact of Smoking on COPD

Smoking is the leading cause of Chronic Obstructive Pulmonary Disease (COPD) and continuing to smoke after a diagnosis can accelerate the progression of the disease. Quitting smoking is the single most effective action a COPD patient can take to halt further lung damage, improve lung function, and enhance overall health.

Why Quitting Can Be Challenging

Nicotine addiction makes quitting smoking a significant challenge for many. The habit is often deeply ingrained in daily routines, serving as a response to stress or a social activity. Withdrawal symptoms can include irritability, cravings, anxiety, depression, and weight gain, making the process difficult but not insurmountable.

Effective Strategies for Quitting Smoking

- **Set a Quit Date:** Choose a quit date a few weeks in advance to prepare mentally and physically. Avoid dates where you expect high stress.

- **Identify Triggers:** Recognize situations, emotions, or activities that increase the urge to smoke. Plan strategies to avoid or manage these triggers without smoking.

- **Use Nicotine Replacement Therapy (NRT):** Products like patches, gum, lozenges, inhalers, or nasal sprays can help manage withdrawal symptoms by delivering small, controlled amounts of nicotine without the harmful chemicals found in cigarettes.

- **Consider Prescription Medications:** Certain medications can reduce cravings and withdrawal symptoms. Talk to a healthcare provider about options like varenicline or bupropion.

- **Seek Behavioral Support:** Counseling, support groups, or quitline services can provide guidance, encouragement, and coping strategies. Combining behavioral support with pharmacotherapy increases the chances of success.

- **Practice Stress Management:** Explore healthy ways to manage stress, such as exercise, meditation, deep breathing, or hobbies.

- **Leverage Technology:** Mobile apps and online programs designed to support quitting smoking can offer daily tips, tracking, and encouragement.

- **Inform Friends and Family:** Share your plan to quit with friends and family. Their support can make a significant difference in overcoming challenges.

- **Reward Progress:** Set milestones and reward yourself for reaching them. This can help reinforce your commitment and celebrate achievements without smoking.

Dealing with Relapses

Relapse is a common part of the quitting process. If you do smoke after your quit date, don't view it as a failure. Instead, analyze what led to the relapse and use it as a learning opportunity to strengthen your quit plan. Remember, every attempt at quitting brings you closer to success.

Conclusion

Quitting smoking is essential for managing COPD effectively. While it may be challenging, the benefits for lung health and overall well-being are undeniable. With the right combination of strategies, support, and treatments, achieving a smoke-free life is possible, leading to significant improvements in the quality and longevity of life for individuals with COPD.

5.4 Exercise: 10 MCQs with Answers at the End

Test your knowledge on lifestyle modifications and COPD management with these multiple-choice questions. Answers are provided at the end for self-assessment.

1. What is the primary benefit of quitting smoking for individuals with COPD?

   A. Immediate lung function improvement

   B. Halting further lung damage

   C. Complete recovery of lung health

   D. Elimination of the need for medication

2. Which dietary approach is recommended for COPD patients experiencing unintentional weight loss?

   A. Low-carbohydrate diet

   B. High-protein, energy-dense foods

   C. Calorie restriction

   D. Intermittent fasting

3. Aerobic exercises for COPD patients include:

A. Heavy weightlifting

B. High-intensity interval training

C. Walking and cycling

D. Breath holding exercises

4. The use of nicotine replacement therapy (NRT) helps by:

A. Delivering small, controlled amounts of nicotine

B. Increasing lung capacity

C. Providing an immediate cure for COPD

D. Enhancing the flavor of food

5. Which of the following is NOT a common withdrawal symptom of quitting smoking?

A. Irritability

B. Enhanced lung function

C. Cravings for nicotine

D. Weight gain

6. Behavioral support for quitting smoking can include:

A. Avoiding physical activity

B. Increasing caffeine intake

C. Counseling or support groups

D. Starting a new smoking habit

7. The primary role of pulmonary rehabilitation in COPD management is to:

A. Replace the need for medications

B. Train patients for lung surgery

C. Improve physical and emotional well-being

D. Increase dependency on oxygen therapy

8. Effective stress management techniques for COPD patients might include:

A. Starting smoking again to reduce stress

B. Practicing meditation and deep breathing

C. Avoiding all forms of exercise

D. Increasing daily nicotine intake

9. For COPD patients who are overweight, the recommended dietary adjustment is:

A. Unrestricted fat intake

B. High sodium diet

C. Balanced diet with controlled portion sizes

D. Exclusive focus on protein intake

10. Relapse in the context of quitting smoking should be viewed as:

    A. A failure that cannot be overcome

    B. An expected part of the quitting process

    C. A sign to give up trying to quit

    D. Irrelevant to COPD management

Answers:

1. B. Halting further lung damage

2. B. High-protein, energy-dense foods

3. C. Walking and cycling

4. A. Delivering small, controlled amounts of nicotine

5. B. Enhanced lung function

6. C. Counseling or support groups

7. C. Improve physical and emotional well-being

8. B. Practicing meditation and deep breathing

9. C. Balanced diet with controlled portion sizes

10. B. An expected part of the quitting process

Chapter 6: Advanced COPD Care

6.1 Oxygen Therapy: Understanding the Basics

The Role of Oxygen Therapy in COPD

For individuals with advanced Chronic Obstructive Pulmonary Disease (COPD), maintaining adequate oxygen levels can become increasingly difficult. Oxygen therapy is prescribed to supplement the body's oxygen needs, improve quality of life, and, in some cases, extend survival. It is typically recommended for patients with severe COPD who have low levels of oxygen in their blood (hypoxemia).

Types of Oxygen Therapy

- **Long-term Oxygen Therapy (LTOT):** Used for patients who need supplemental oxygen for many hours each day, often including during sleep and sometimes 24 hours a day.

- **Short-burst Oxygen Therapy:** Used to relieve sudden episodes of breathlessness, not typically recommended for long-term management of COPD.

- **Ambulatory Oxygen:** Designed for use when the patient is active or moving around, helping to maintain an active lifestyle.

Delivery Systems for Oxygen Therapy

- **Oxygen Concentrators:** Devices that extract oxygen from room air, providing a continuous supply. They are suitable for use at home and can be adjusted to deliver the required flow rate of oxygen.

- **Compressed Oxygen Tanks/Cylinders:** Portable tanks that contain oxygen gas, useful for people who are active outside their homes.

- **Liquid Oxygen Systems:** Contain oxygen in liquid form, which converts to gas before inhalation. These systems can be more compact and last longer than gas cylinders, making them convenient for ambulatory use.

Benefits of Oxygen Therapy

- **Improved Survival:** LTOT, particularly when used for more than 15 hours a day, has been shown to improve survival rates in patients with severe, resting hypoxemia.

- **Enhanced Exercise Tolerance:** Supplemental oxygen can improve the ability to participate in physical activities by reducing breathlessness.

- **Better Quality of Life:** Oxygen therapy can help alleviate symptoms of hypoxemia, such as fatigue and cognitive impairment, leading to an overall improvement in quality of life.

Considerations and Safety Tips

- **Regular Monitoring:** Oxygen therapy requires regular monitoring by healthcare providers to ensure oxygen levels are kept within a safe range.

- **Avoiding Fire Hazards:** Oxygen supports combustion, so it's important to avoid open flames, smoking, and flammable materials when using oxygen therapy.

- **Travel and Mobility:** Patients using oxygen therapy need to plan for travel and mobility, considering the portability of their oxygen supply and any additional requirements for air travel.

Conclusion

Oxygen therapy is a crucial component of advanced COPD care, offering significant benefits for patients with severe hypoxemia. By improving oxygen levels, this therapy can enhance exercise tolerance, quality of life, and survival. Successful oxygen therapy requires careful management and adherence to safety precautions, ensuring that patients receive the maximum possible benefit.

6.2 Ventilatory Support for Severe COPD

Understanding Ventilatory Support

For patients with severe Chronic Obstructive Pulmonary Disease (COPD) and advanced respiratory failure, ventilatory support may become necessary. This intervention helps alleviate the workload of breathing, improves gas exchange, and supports the respiratory muscles, potentially enhancing both quality of life and survival.

Types of Ventilatory Support

- **Non-invasive Ventilation (NIV):** NIV is a common form of ventilatory support for COPD patients, typically delivered through a mask that covers the nose, the mouth, or both. It includes Continuous Positive Airway Pressure (CPAP) and Bilevel Positive Airway Pressure (BiPAP). BiPAP is particularly beneficial as it provides two levels of pressure: higher pressure when the patient inhales and lower pressure during exhalation.

- **Invasive Mechanical Ventilation:** In severe cases, particularly during acute exacerbations leading to respiratory failure, invasive mechanical ventilation may be required. This involves intubation through the mouth or a tracheostomy and is performed in a hospital setting.

Benefits of Ventilatory Support

- **Improved Blood Gas Levels:** Ventilatory support helps correct hypoxemia (low blood oxygen levels) and hypercapnia (high blood carbon dioxide levels), stabilizing the patient's condition.

- **Reduced Respiratory Effort:** By assisting or fully taking over the work of breathing, ventilatory support allows the respiratory muscles to rest and recover, reducing fatigue and breathlessness.

- **Enhanced Sleep Quality:** NIV, particularly at night, can improve sleep quality and efficiency, addressing issues like sleep apnea that are common in severe COPD.

- **Increased Exercise Capacity:** With improved breathing support, patients may find it easier to participate in pulmonary rehabilitation and daily activities, enhancing their overall functional status.

Considerations for Ventilatory Support

- **Patient Selection:** Not all COPD patients are candidates for ventilatory support. It's typically considered for those with advanced disease, repeated exacerbations, or chronic respiratory failure.

- **Adherence and Comfort:** The success of NIV largely depends on the patient's comfort and adherence to the treatment. Proper mask fit and gradual acclimatization to the device are crucial.

- **Monitoring and Adjustments:** Regular monitoring by healthcare professionals is necessary to ensure the effectiveness of ventilatory support, with adjustments made based on the patient's response and changes in their condition.

- **End-of-life Considerations:** Invasive mechanical ventilation may be used in acute, life-threatening situations. Discussions about the goals of care, including advanced directives and the use of life-sustaining treatments, are important aspects of managing severe COPD.

Conclusion

Ventilatory support offers significant benefits for patients with severe COPD, potentially improving survival, reducing symptoms, and enhancing quality of life. Whether through non-invasive or invasive means, careful consideration of the patient's overall health status, preferences, and goals of care is essential to optimize outcomes and ensure that ventilatory support aligns with the individual's needs and wishes.

6.3 Palliative Care and End-of-Life Considerations

Palliative Care in COPD Management

Palliative care is a specialized area of healthcare that focuses on relieving and preventing the suffering of patients. For those with severe Chronic Obstructive Pulmonary Disease (COPD), palliative care aims to improve quality of life by addressing physical symptoms, emotional stress, and spiritual concerns associated with the disease and its progression.

Key Components of Palliative Care for COPD

- **Symptom Management:** Efforts are directed towards managing distressing symptoms such as dyspnea (shortness of breath), chronic cough, fatigue, and pain, using medications, oxygen therapy, and non-pharmacological methods like breathing techniques.

- **Psychological and Emotional Support:** Palliative care provides support for anxiety, depression, and other emotional aspects of living with COPD, including individual counseling and support groups.

- **Advance Care Planning:** Discussions about advance directives, such as living wills and health care proxy designations, ensure that the patient's preferences for treatment and end-of-life care are understood and respected.

- **Caregiver Support:** Palliative care also extends to family members and caregivers, offering them resources, respite care, and counseling to help manage the stresses of caregiving.

End-of-Life Considerations

As COPD progresses to its advanced stages, discussions about end-of-life care become increasingly important. These conversations can be challenging but are essential for ensuring that care aligns with the patient's values and wishes.

- **Hospice Care:** For patients in the final stages of COPD who choose to focus on comfort rather than aggressive treatment, hospice care provides comprehensive symptom management, emotional support, and spiritual care in the patient's home or a hospice facility.

- **Decision Making:** Decisions may include the use of ventilatory support, preferences for hospitalization during exacerbations, and the initiation or withdrawal of life-sustaining treatments.

- **Communication:** Open, honest communication between patients, families, and healthcare providers is crucial in navigating the complexities of end-of-life care, ensuring that decisions are made collaboratively and respectfully.

The Role of the Healthcare Team

The management of severe COPD at the end of life requires a multidisciplinary approach. Pulmonologists, primary care providers, palliative care specialists, nurses, social workers, and spiritual care providers work together to address the comprehensive needs of the patient and family.

Conclusion

Palliative care and end-of-life considerations are integral components of managing severe COPD. By focusing on symptom relief, emotional support, and respecting patient preferences, palliative care seeks to enhance the quality of life for patients and their families during the challenging stages of the disease. Encouraging early discussions about palliative care options and advance care planning can facilitate a more personalized and compassionate approach to care at the end of life.

6.4 Exercise: 10 MCQs with Answers at the End

Assess your understanding of advanced COPD care, including oxygen therapy, ventilatory support, palliative care, and end-of-life considerations, with these multiple-choice questions. Answers are provided at the end for self-assessment.

1. What is the primary goal of oxygen therapy in severe COPD?

A. To cure COPD

B. To improve oxygen saturation

C. To reduce carbon dioxide levels

D. To increase physical strength

2. Non-invasive ventilation (NIV) is mainly indicated for COPD patients with:

A. Mild COPD

B. Severe COPD and chronic respiratory failure

C. COPD and lung cancer

D. Early-stage COPD

3. The primary benefit of palliative care in COPD is to:

A. Provide a cure for COPD

B. Delay the progression of COPD

C. Improve the quality of life

D. Increase lung capacity

4. Advance care planning in COPD includes discussions about:

A. Exercise routines

B. Vacation plans

C. End-of-life care preferences

D. Dietary supplements

5. Which of the following is NOT a component of palliative care for COPD?

   A. Aggressive fluid resuscitation

   B. Symptom management

   C. Psychological support

   D. Advance care planning

6. Long-term oxygen therapy (LTOT) has been shown to improve:

   A. Exercise tolerance in mild COPD

   B. Survival in patients with severe resting hypoxemia

   C. Cognitive function in healthy adults

   D. Lung function in asthma

7. Ventilatory support for severe COPD may include:

   A. Oral medications only

   B. Invasive and non-invasive ventilation

   C. Surgery as a first option

   D. Avoiding oxygen use

8. Hospice care for COPD focuses on:

A. Aggressive treatment to extend life

B. Comfort and quality of life at the end of life

C. Introducing new treatments for COPD

D. Rehabilitation exercises

9. Effective symptom management in advanced COPD can include:

A. Limiting fluid intake to reduce cough

B. Using oxygen therapy to relieve breathlessness

C. Completely avoiding the use of inhalers

D. Increasing exposure to outdoor pollution

10. Palliative care for COPD patients is best initiated:

A. Only in the final days before death

B. After all other treatments have failed

C. Early in the course of the disease to manage symptoms effectively

D. When the patient requests it, and not before

Answers:

1. B. To improve oxygen saturation

2. B. Severe COPD and chronic respiratory failure

3. C. Improve the quality of life

4. C. End-of-life care preferences

5. A. Aggressive fluid resuscitation

6. B. Survival in patients with severe resting hypoxemia

7. B. Invasive and non-invasive ventilation

8. B. Comfort and quality of life at the end of life

9. B. Using oxygen therapy to relieve breathlessness

10. C. Early in the course of the disease to manage symptoms effectively

Chapter 7: Preventing COPD Exacerbations

7.1 Identifying and Avoiding Triggers

The Importance of Managing Exacerbations

Chronic Obstructive Pulmonary Disease (COPD) exacerbations are periods when symptoms become significantly worse than the daily baseline and can have a profound impact on patients' health and quality of life. Preventing these exacerbations is crucial, as they can lead to a rapid decline in lung function, increased hospitalizations, and even death. A key strategy in managing COPD and reducing the risk of exacerbations is identifying and avoiding known triggers.

Common Triggers of COPD Exacerbations

- **Tobacco Smoke:** Smoke from cigarettes, cigars, and pipes is a major irritant that can worsen COPD symptoms and trigger exacerbations. Avoiding smoking and secondhand smoke is essential.

- **Air Pollution:** Outdoor air pollutants (e.g., car exhaust, industrial emissions) and indoor pollutants (e.g., cooking fumes, chemical vapors from cleaning products) can irritate the lungs and exacerbate COPD.

- **Respiratory Infections:** Viruses that cause colds and flu can lead to severe exacerbations. Bacterial infections can also be problematic. Annual flu vaccinations, good hand hygiene, and avoiding close contact with sick individuals are preventive measures.

- **Weather Changes:** Extreme temperatures (both hot and cold) and sudden weather changes can trigger symptoms. Staying indoors during very cold or hot weather and using air conditioning or heating appropriately can help.

- **Allergens:** Pollen, mold, dust mites, and pet dander can provoke COPD symptoms. Reducing exposure to these allergens by keeping the living environment clean and using air purifiers can be beneficial.

- **Physical Exertion:** While regular, moderate exercise is beneficial for COPD patients, overexertion can sometimes trigger an exacerbation. Tailoring exercise intensity to individual capabilities is important.

- **Stress and Emotional Upsets:** Stress can worsen COPD symptoms, potentially leading to exacerbations. Techniques such as mindfulness, relaxation exercises, and counseling can help manage stress.

Strategies to Avoid Triggers

- **Environmental Control:** Use air purifiers, maintain a clean home, avoid outdoor activities on high pollution days, and ensure good ventilation to reduce exposure to indoor and outdoor pollutants.

- **Lifestyle Modifications:** Quit smoking, avoid areas where smoking occurs, and practice good nutrition and regular exercise within personal limits.

- **Infection Prevention:** Stay up to date with vaccinations, practice good hand hygiene, and avoid crowded places during flu season.

- **Education:** Understanding COPD and being aware of personal triggers are key. Patients should be educated on recognizing early signs of exacerbations and how to act promptly.

Conclusion

Preventing COPD exacerbations involves a comprehensive approach centered on identifying and avoiding triggers. Through environmental control, lifestyle modifications, infection prevention, and education, individuals with COPD can achieve better disease management, improve their quality of life, and potentially reduce the risk of severe exacerbations.

7.2 Vaccinations and Preventive Measures

Vaccinations: A Key Strategy in COPD Management

Vaccinations play a vital role in the management of Chronic Obstructive Pulmonary Disease (COPD) by protecting against respiratory infections that can lead to exacerbations and further compromise lung function. Immunizations recommended for individuals with COPD are designed to prevent infections that are particularly dangerous for people with chronic lung conditions.

Recommended Vaccinations for COPD Patients

- **Influenza Vaccine:** An annual flu shot is recommended for all COPD patients. The influenza virus can cause severe respiratory infections, leading to hospitalization and significant complications in individuals with COPD. The flu vaccine reduces the risk of illness and exacerbations associated with the flu.

- **Pneumococcal Vaccine:** This vaccine protects against pneumococcal disease, including pneumonia, meningitis, and bloodstream infections caused by the Streptococcus pneumoniae bacteria. Two types of pneumococcal vaccines are recommended for adults with COPD: Pneumococcal Conjugate Vaccine (PCV13 or PCV15, depending on the country's guidelines) and Pneumococcal Polysaccharide Vaccine (PPSV23), administered in a sequence recommended by healthcare providers.

- **COVID-19 Vaccine:** The COVID-19 pandemic has highlighted the importance of vaccination in protecting vulnerable populations, including those with COPD. COVID-19 vaccines are recommended to prevent severe illness, hospitalizations, and death caused by the SARS-CoV-2 virus.

- **Tdap Vaccine:** The Tdap vaccine protects against tetanus, diphtheria, and pertussis (whooping cough). A one-time dose is recommended for adults, including those with COPD, followed by a Td (tetanus and diphtheria) booster every 10 years.

Additional Preventive Measures

Besides vaccination, COPD patients can take several other preventive measures to reduce the risk of respiratory infections:

- **Hand Hygiene:** Regular handwashing with soap and water or the use of alcohol-based hand sanitizers can significantly reduce the spread of infectious agents.

- **Avoiding Crowds:** Especially during flu season or outbreaks of respiratory illnesses, avoiding crowded places can help reduce the risk of catching infections.

- **Healthy Lifestyle:** A balanced diet, regular exercise, and adequate sleep strengthen the immune system, making it better equipped to fight infections.

- **Smoking Cessation:** Quitting smoking is the most effective step COPD patients can take to slow the progression of their disease and reduce the risk of infections.

- **Wearing Masks:** In certain situations, such as during outbreaks of respiratory infections, wearing masks can provide additional protection against airborne pathogens.

Conclusion

Vaccinations are a cornerstone of preventive care for individuals with COPD, effectively reducing the risk of serious respiratory infections and their complications. Along with other preventive measures, vaccinations contribute to better disease management, fewer exacerbations, and improved overall health outcomes for COPD patients. Healthcare providers play a crucial role in educating patients about the benefits of vaccines and implementing comprehensive vaccination strategies tailored to individual needs.

7.3 Managing Comorbidities

The Challenge of Comorbidities in COPD

Chronic Obstructive Pulmonary Disease (COPD) often does not occur in isolation; it is frequently accompanied by other chronic conditions, known as comorbidities, which can complicate the management of COPD and affect overall health and quality of life. Proper management of these comorbidities is crucial for optimizing COPD care and improving patient outcomes.

Common Comorbidities in COPD Patients

- **Cardiovascular Diseases:** Conditions like hypertension, heart failure, and coronary artery disease are more common in individuals with COPD. The systemic inflammation associated with COPD can contribute to cardiovascular risk.

- **Osteoporosis:** The combination of chronic inflammation, steroid use, and reduced physical activity can increase the risk of bone density loss and fractures.

- **Diabetes Mellitus:** There is a higher prevalence of type 2 diabetes in individuals with COPD, potentially due to shared risk factors like smoking and physical inactivity.

- **Anxiety and Depression:** The limitations imposed by COPD can lead to feelings of isolation and frustration, increasing the risk of mental health issues.

- **Lung Cancer:** Smoking is a common risk factor for both COPD and lung cancer, making lung cancer more prevalent among individuals with COPD.

Strategies for Managing Comorbidities

- **Comprehensive Assessment:** Regular screening for common comorbidities allows for early detection and intervention. Healthcare providers should adopt a holistic approach to patient care, considering the interplay between COPD and other conditions.

- **Integrated Care Plans:** Management plans should be tailored to address both COPD and its comorbidities. For example, optimizing cardiovascular health can improve respiratory outcomes, and vice versa.

- **Medication Management:** It's essential to review all medications regularly to avoid potential interactions and ensure they do not exacerbate other conditions. For instance, certain beta-blockers used for heart disease can affect lung function but cardio-selective beta-blockers may be safer for COPD patients.

- **Lifestyle Modifications:** Smoking cessation, regular physical activity, a balanced diet, and weight management are critical components of managing both COPD and many of its comorbidities.

- **Mental Health Support:** Providing access to mental health services, including counseling and support groups, can help address the psychological aspects of living with COPD and comorbid conditions.

- **Patient Education:** Empowering patients with knowledge about their conditions, treatment options, and lifestyle changes that can mitigate risk factors is vital for effective comorbidity management.

Conclusion

Managing comorbidities in COPD requires a coordinated, multidisciplinary approach that addresses the full spectrum of a patient's health needs. By recognizing and treating comorbid conditions, healthcare providers can significantly enhance the quality of care for individuals with COPD, leading to better health outcomes, reduced hospitalizations, and an improved quality of life.

7.4 Exercise: 10 MCQs with Answers at the End

Test your understanding of preventing COPD exacerbations, including strategies for identifying and avoiding triggers, the importance of vaccinations, managing comorbidities, and other preventive measures with these multiple-choice questions. Answers are provided at the end for self-assessment.

1. What is the most effective way to prevent COPD exacerbations related to smoking?

   A. Smoking low-tar cigarettes

   B. Using air purifiers at home

   C. Quitting smoking

   D. Smoking only outdoors

2. Which vaccination is NOT typically recommended for patients with COPD?

   A. Influenza vaccine

   B. Pneumococcal vaccine

   C. COVID-19 vaccine

   D. Varicella vaccine

3. Managing which comorbidity can significantly impact the management of COPD?

A. Osteoporosis

B. Hypertension

C. Both A and B

D. Neither A nor B

4. What is a common trigger of COPD exacerbations that can be controlled indoors?

A. Pollen

B. Indoor air pollutants

C. Extreme temperatures

D. Emotional stress

5. Which of the following is a benefit of regular exercise for COPD patients?

A. Increased lung capacity

B. Reduced risk of exacerbations

C. Immediate cessation of symptoms

D. Complete recovery from COPD

6. How can weather changes trigger COPD exacerbations?

    A. By causing air pressure changes only

    B. Through temperature extremes and humidity changes

    C. By improving air quality

    D. Weather changes do not affect COPD

7. Why is mental health support important for COPD patients?

    A. It can improve lung function directly

    B. It addresses comorbid conditions like anxiety and depression

    C. It eliminates the need for medication

    D. It reduces the frequency of respiratory infections

8. What role do vaccinations play in COPD management?

    A. They cure COPD

    B. They directly improve lung function

    C. They prevent infections that could lead to exacerbations

    D. They reduce the need for oxygen therapy

9. Which lifestyle modification is crucial for managing COPD and its comorbidities?

    A. High-intensity interval training

    B. Following a high-fat diet

    C. Smoking cessation

D. Avoiding all physical activity

10. How does avoiding crowds benefit COPD patients?

A. It increases physical activity

B. It reduces the risk of respiratory infections

C. It eliminates the need for vaccinations

D. It directly improves lung function

Answers:

1. C. Quitting smoking

2. D. Varicella vaccine

3. C. Both A and B

4. B. Indoor air pollutants

5. B. Reduced risk of exacerbations

6. B. Through temperature extremes and humidity changes

7. B. It addresses comorbid conditions like anxiety and depression

8. C. They prevent infections that could lead to exacerbations

9. C. Smoking cessation

10. B. It reduces the risk of respiratory infections

Chapter 8: The Role of Technology in COPD Management

8.1 Telemedicine and Remote Monitoring

Embracing Technology in COPD Care

The integration of technology into healthcare has transformed the management of Chronic Obstructive Pulmonary Disease (COPD), offering innovative ways to monitor and support patients remotely. Telemedicine and remote monitoring have emerged as pivotal tools, enabling continuous care and improving patient outcomes while reducing the need for in-person visits.

Telemedicine: Bridging the Gap

Telemedicine allows patients and healthcare providers to communicate using digital platforms, facilitating virtual consultations, and follow-ups. This approach is particularly beneficial for COPD management for several reasons:

- **Accessibility:** Patients living in remote areas or with mobility issues can easily access specialist care.

- **Convenience:** Reduces the need for travel, saving time and resources for both patients and healthcare providers.

- **Early Intervention:** Enables timely management advice, potentially preventing exacerbations and hospital admissions.

- **Education and Support:** Provides a platform for patient education, promoting self-management skills and offering psychological support.

Remote Monitoring: Keeping a Close Eye

Remote monitoring involves the use of devices and applications to collect and transmit health data from patients to their healthcare providers in real time or periodically. This data can include vital signs, oxygen levels, and symptoms related to COPD. Key benefits include:

- **Real-time Data Collection:** Allows for the continuous monitoring of a patient's condition, enabling swift adjustments to treatment plans as needed.

- **Exacerbation Detection:** Early signs of exacerbations can be detected, allowing for prompt intervention.

- **Medication Adherence:** Some systems remind patients to take their medications and track adherence.

- **Lifestyle Modification:** Can encourage and monitor lifestyle changes, such as increased physical activity.

Implementing Telemedicine and Remote Monitoring

Successful implementation requires consideration of several factors:

- **Technology Access and Literacy:** Patients need access to the necessary technology and must be comfortable using it. Training sessions can be beneficial.

- **Privacy and Security:** Ensuring the confidentiality and security of patient data is paramount.

- **Integration with Care Plans:** Technology should complement existing care plans, not replace the essential elements of traditional care.

- **Personalization:** Tailoring technology use to individual patient needs and preferences can enhance engagement and effectiveness.

Conclusion

Telemedicine and remote monitoring represent significant advancements in COPD management, offering numerous benefits for patient care, education, and support. By facilitating better access to healthcare providers, enabling real-time health monitoring, and supporting self-management, technology can play a crucial role in improving the quality of life for individuals with COPD. As technology evolves, its integration into COPD care is expected to deepen, further enhancing patient outcomes and healthcare efficiency.

8.2 Wearable Technology for Lung Health

Innovations in Monitoring Respiratory Conditions

Wearable technology has rapidly evolved, becoming a key player in monitoring and managing health conditions, including Chronic Obstructive Pulmonary Disease (COPD). These devices, ranging from smartwatches to chest straps, offer continuous, real-time monitoring of various health metrics relevant to lung health and COPD management.

Types of Wearable Technology for COPD

- **Smartwatches and Fitness Trackers:** These devices can monitor heart rate, activity levels, and even oxygen saturation (SpO2), providing insights into the patient's physical activity and overall health status.

- **Chest Straps and Sensors:** Specifically designed for respiratory monitoring, these wearables can track breathing patterns, respiratory rate, and effort, alerting patients to potential exacerbations or the need for medication adjustments.

- **Wearable Spirometers:** Compact and portable, these devices allow patients to perform regular spirometry tests at home, tracking lung function over time and detecting changes that may indicate a need for intervention.

Benefits of Wearable Technology for COPD Management

- **Early Detection of Exacerbations:** By monitoring trends in respiratory metrics, wearables can help identify early signs of exacerbations, allowing for prompt treatment and potentially avoiding hospitalization.

- **Improved Self-Management:** Access to real-time data empowers patients to better understand their condition, recognize triggers, and make informed decisions about their health.

- **Enhanced Physical Activity:** Activity trackers encourage patients to maintain or increase their level of physical activity, which is crucial for managing COPD and improving quality of life.

- **Remote Monitoring and Telehealth Integration:** Data collected by wearables can be shared with healthcare providers, enhancing remote monitoring capabilities and integrating seamlessly with telehealth services for comprehensive care management.

Considerations for Implementing Wearable Technology

- **Accuracy and Reliability:** It's essential to choose devices that are clinically validated for accuracy, especially for critical measurements like oxygen saturation.

- **User-Friendliness:** Devices should be easy to use and interpret by patients, regardless of their technological proficiency.

- **Cost and Accessibility:** Consideration should be given to the cost of these technologies and their accessibility to all patients, including those with limited financial resources.

- **Data Privacy:** Ensuring the privacy and security of health data collected by wearables is paramount to maintaining patient trust and compliance with regulations.

Conclusion

Wearable technology offers promising benefits for the management of COPD, providing valuable insights into lung health and enabling proactive care strategies. As these technologies continue to advance, their integration into standard COPD care practices could significantly enhance patient outcomes, improve quality of life, and reduce the burden on healthcare systems. However, careful consideration of their limitations and challenges is essential to maximize their potential benefits.

8.3 Apps and Digital Tools for Self-Management

Leveraging Digital Solutions in COPD Care

In the digital age, mobile applications and digital tools have become invaluable for managing chronic conditions like Chronic Obstructive Pulmonary Disease (COPD). These platforms offer patients the means to actively participate in their care, track their condition, and access educational resources at their fingertips, fostering an informed and proactive approach to managing COPD.

Key Features of COPD Management Apps

- **Symptom Tracking:** Users can log daily symptoms, medication use, and triggers, helping them and their healthcare providers identify patterns and adjust treatment plans accordingly.

- **Medication Reminders:** To ensure adherence to medication schedules, apps can send reminders to users, reducing the risk of missed doses and exacerbations.

- **Pulmonary Rehabilitation Exercises:** Some apps provide guided exercises and breathing techniques to improve lung function and overall fitness.

- **Educational Resources:** Access to reliable information about COPD, including tips for managing symptoms, dietary recommendations, and strategies for quitting smoking.

- **Progress Monitoring:** Features that allow users to track improvements in their symptoms and quality of life over time, offering motivation and positive reinforcement.

- **Telehealth Integration:** The ability to share data collected through the app with healthcare providers during virtual consultations, enhancing the quality of telemedicine visits.

Benefits of Using Apps and Digital Tools for COPD

- **Empowered Self-Management:** Equipped with the right tools and information, patients can take an active role in managing their COPD, leading to improved outcomes.

- **Early Intervention:** By facilitating the early detection of worsening symptoms or exacerbations, apps can prompt timely medical intervention, potentially averting hospital admissions.

- **Enhanced Patient-Provider Communication:** Digital tools can streamline communication between patients and their healthcare team, ensuring that care decisions are informed by comprehensive, real-time data.

- **Improved Adherence:** Medication reminders and educational resources can improve adherence to treatment plans and lifestyle recommendations, key components of effective COPD management.

Considerations for Choosing and Using COPD Apps

- **Clinical Validation:** Opt for apps that have been developed with input from healthcare professionals and, ideally, validated through clinical research.

- **User Privacy:** Ensure that the app has a clear privacy policy detailing how personal health information is protected.

- **Customization:** The ability to customize features according to individual needs and preferences can enhance the user experience and engagement.

- **Regular Updates:** Apps should be regularly updated based on user feedback and the latest COPD research to ensure they remain relevant and useful.

Conclusion

Apps and digital tools for self-management offer promising support for individuals with COPD, complementing traditional care methods and empowering patients with the knowledge and resources to manage their condition effectively. As technology continues to evolve, the potential for these tools to improve the quality of life for COPD patients is immense, signaling a shift towards more personalized, patient-centered care models.

8.4 Exercise: 10 MCQs with Answers at the End

Test your understanding of the role of technology in COPD management, including telemedicine, wearable technology, apps, and digital tools for self-management, with these multiple-choice questions. Answers are provided at the end for self-assessment.

1. What is a primary benefit of telemedicine in managing COPD?

   A. It replaces the need for medication.

B. It allows for physical examinations.

C. It enables remote consultations and monitoring.

D. It cures COPD.

2. How do wearable technologies benefit COPD patients?

A. By providing continuous, real-time health data monitoring.

B. By increasing lung capacity.

C. By filtering the air breathed by the patient.

D. By delivering oxygen therapy.

3. What type of app feature is beneficial for ensuring COPD patients adhere to their medication schedule?

A. Game-based challenges.

B. Medication reminders.

C. Social media integration.

D. Weather updates.

4. Which of the following is NOT a direct benefit of using apps and digital tools for COPD management?

A. Cure for COPD.

B. Symptom tracking.

C. Access to educational resources.

D. Pulmonary rehabilitation exercises.

5. Remote monitoring devices for COPD patients can track all the following EXCEPT:

A. Oxygen levels.

B. Respiratory rate.

C. Lung capacity changes over time.

D. Blood glucose levels.

6. Telemedicine can improve COPD management through:

A. Eliminating the need for hospital visits.

B. Reducing physical activity.

C. Timely intervention based on symptom monitoring.

D. Providing a platform for surgical procedures.

7. Wearable spirometers are used for:

A. Delivering medications.

B. Monitoring lung function over time.

C. Filtering harmful pollutants from the air.

D. Providing non-invasive ventilation.

8. COPD management apps can help patients by:

A. Offering guided breathing exercises.

B. Serving as a substitute for oxygen therapy.

C. Predicting weather changes.

D. Automatically adjusting CPAP machines.

9. Which of the following is a consideration when choosing a COPD management app?

A. Celebrity endorsements.

B. The number of downloads.

C. Clinical validation and user privacy.

D. Availability of in-app purchases.

10. The integration of technology into COPD care primarily aims to:

A. Completely replace traditional healthcare.

B. Facilitate self-management and enhance care.

C. Discourage physical visits to healthcare providers.

D. Promote a technology-only approach to treatment.

Answers:

1. C. It enables remote consultations and monitoring.

2. A. By providing continuous, real-time health data monitoring.

3. B. Medication reminders.

4. A. Cure for COPD.

5. D. Blood glucose levels.

6. C. Timely intervention based on symptom monitoring.

7. B. Monitoring lung function over time.

8. A. Offering guided breathing exercises.

9. C. Clinical validation and user privacy.

10. B. Facilitate self-management and enhance care.

Chapter 9: The Psychological Impact of COPD

9.1 Coping with Chronic Illness

Understanding the Psychological Challenges

Living with Chronic Obstructive Pulmonary Disease (COPD) poses significant psychological challenges. The chronic nature of the disease, the progressive loss of lung function, and the limitations on daily activities can lead to emotional distress, impacting mental health and overall quality of life. Coping with these challenges requires resilience, support, and effective strategies to maintain mental well-being.

Common Psychological Responses

- **Anxiety and Depression:** The fear of breathlessness and the uncertainty about the future can lead to anxiety, while the loss of independence and changes in lifestyle can trigger depression.

- **Stress:** Managing the symptoms of COPD, along with the potential financial burdens and changes in family dynamics, can contribute to chronic stress.

- **Isolation and Loneliness:** Physical limitations might lead to reduced social interactions, causing feelings of isolation and loneliness.

Strategies for Coping with COPD

- **Seek Professional Help:** Consulting with mental health professionals can provide coping strategies for dealing with anxiety, depression, and stress. Cognitive-behavioral therapy (CBT) has been shown to be particularly effective.

- **Participate in Support Groups:** COPD support groups offer a platform to share experiences and strategies, reducing feelings of isolation. Connecting with others who understand the challenges of living with COPD can be incredibly supportive.

- **Educate Yourself and Others:** Understanding COPD and its implications can help in managing the disease more effectively. Educating family and friends about COPD can also garner more understanding and support.

- **Develop Healthy Habits:** Regular physical activity, balanced nutrition, and adequate rest can improve physical health, which in turn can positively impact mental health.

- **Practice Mindfulness and Relaxation Techniques:** Techniques such as deep breathing, meditation, and progressive muscle relaxation can help manage stress and anxiety.

 - **Set Realistic Goals:** Setting achievable goals can provide a sense of purpose and accomplishment, boosting self-esteem and motivation.

- **Focus on What You Can Control:** Accepting the diagnosis and focusing on aspects of life that can be controlled, such as treatment adherence and lifestyle changes, can help maintain a positive outlook.

The Role of Healthcare Providers

Healthcare providers play a crucial role in identifying psychological distress in COPD patients and providing referrals to appropriate mental health services. Incorporating mental health assessments into routine COPD care can ensure that patients receive the support they need to cope with the disease effectively.

Conclusion

Coping with the psychological impact of COPD is an integral part of managing the disease. By adopting effective coping strategies, seeking support, and focusing on maintaining mental and physical health, individuals with COPD can lead fulfilling lives despite the challenges posed by the illness. Healthcare providers, support networks, and the patients themselves must work together to address the psychological aspects of COPD, ensuring comprehensive care that goes beyond physical symptoms.

9.2 Depression and Anxiety in COPD Patients

The Psychological Burden of COPD

Depression and anxiety are significantly more prevalent among individuals with Chronic Obstructive Pulmonary Disease (COPD) compared to the general population. The physical limitations, chronic nature of the disease, and the fear of exacerbations contribute to a heightened risk of developing these mental health conditions, which can further impact the course of COPD and the patient's quality of life.

Understanding Depression and Anxiety in COPD

- **Depression:** COPD patients may experience persistent sadness, loss of interest in activities, feelings of worthlessness, changes in appetite or weight, and thoughts of death or suicide.

- **Anxiety:** Commonly manifests as persistent worry about health and the future, physical symptoms like increased heart rate and shortness of breath, and panic attacks, which can be particularly distressing when they mimic or worsen COPD symptoms.

Impact on COPD Management

Depression and anxiety can lead to poorer health outcomes in COPD patients by affecting their ability to manage the disease:

- **Reduced Adherence:** Affected patients may be less likely to adhere to treatment plans, perform daily pulmonary rehabilitation exercises, or attend medical appointments.

- **Increased Risk of Exacerbations:** Emotional stress can exacerbate COPD symptoms, leading to more frequent and severe exacerbations.

- **Higher Healthcare Utilization:** Patients with COPD and co-existing depression or anxiety are more likely to have increased hospitalizations and emergency room visits.

Strategies for Managing Depression and Anxiety

- **Professional Mental Health Support:** Psychological counseling, particularly cognitive-behavioral therapy (CBT), can be effective in treating depression and anxiety. In some cases, antidepressant or anti-anxiety medication may be recommended.

- **Pulmonary Rehabilitation:** Participating in pulmonary rehabilitation not only improves physical health but also provides social support and reduces symptoms of depression and anxiety.

- **Social Support:** Engaging with support groups, either in person or online, can reduce feelings of isolation and provide a sense of community.

- **Stress Management Techniques:** Mindfulness, relaxation exercises, and stress management training can help patients cope with anxiety and stress.

- **Regular Physical Activity:** Exercise has been shown to reduce symptoms of depression and anxiety. Tailored exercise programs should be part of the COPD management plan.

Integrating Mental Health Care in COPD Management

Recognizing and treating depression and anxiety in COPD patients is crucial for comprehensive care. Healthcare providers should screen for these conditions regularly and integrate mental health care into the overall management plan, collaborating with mental health professionals to provide holistic care.

Conclusion

Depression and anxiety significantly affect the well-being and management of COPD, highlighting the need for integrated care approaches that address both the physical and psychological aspects of the disease. Through timely diagnosis, targeted interventions, and ongoing support, it is possible to improve the mental health and overall quality of life of individuals living with COPD.

9.3 Support Systems and Counseling

The Importance of Support in COPD Management

Effective management of Chronic Obstructive Pulmonary Disease (COPD) extends beyond medical treatments to include emotional and psychological support. Support systems and counseling play a crucial role in helping patients cope with the challenges of living with a chronic illness, improving their ability to manage the disease, adhere to treatment plans, and maintain a higher quality of life.

Types of Support Systems for COPD Patients

- **Family and Friends:** A strong network of family and friends can provide emotional support, assistance with daily tasks, and encouragement to adhere to treatment and lifestyle changes.

- **COPD Support Groups:** These groups offer a platform for sharing experiences, advice, and coping strategies with others who understand the challenges of living with COPD. Support groups can be found in local communities or online.

  Healthcare Team: Pulmonologists, nurses, respiratory therapists, and other healthcare professionals can provide medical support, education about COPD management, and referrals to additional resources.

The Role of Counseling in COPD Care

- **Individual Counseling:** Professional counseling can help patients address feelings of anxiety, depression, and grief that may accompany a COPD diagnosis. Cognitive-behavioral therapy (CBT) is particularly effective in managing chronic illness-related stress.

- **Family Counseling:** Family members may also experience stress, anxiety, and caregiver burnout. Counseling can help families navigate these challenges, improve communication, and establish healthy coping mechanisms.

- **Pulmonary Rehabilitation Counseling:** Many pulmonary rehabilitation programs include counseling components that focus on lifestyle modifications, stress management, and techniques to manage breathlessness and conserve energy.

Benefits of Support Systems and Counseling

- **Improved Mental Health:** Emotional support and counseling can reduce symptoms of depression and anxiety, leading to improved overall well-being.

- **Enhanced Coping Skills:** Patients learn strategies to cope with the physical and emotional challenges of COPD, helping them to maintain independence and engage in daily activities.

- **Increased Treatment Adherence:** Support from family, peers, and healthcare providers can motivate patients to adhere to their treatment plans, participate in pulmonary rehabilitation, and make beneficial lifestyle changes.

- **Reduced Hospitalizations:** Effective support and counseling can help prevent exacerbations and hospital admissions by promoting better self-management and early intervention for symptoms.

Implementing Support and Counseling in COPD Management

Incorporating support systems and counseling into COPD care requires a multidisciplinary approach. Healthcare providers should routinely assess patients' mental health and social support needs, providing referrals to counseling services and support groups as needed. Encouraging patients to engage with their support networks and participate in counseling can significantly enhance the effectiveness of COPD management.

Conclusion

Support systems and counseling are integral components of comprehensive COPD care. By addressing the emotional and psychological needs of patients and their families, these resources can significantly improve coping strategies, treatment adherence, and overall quality of life for those living with COPD.

9.4 Exercise: 10 MCQs with Answers at the End

Evaluate your understanding of the psychological impact of COPD, including coping mechanisms, the effects of depression and anxiety, the importance of support systems, and the role of counseling, with these multiple-choice questions. Answers are provided at the end for self-assessment.

1. What psychological condition is commonly experienced by individuals with COPD?

   A. Euphoria

   B. Anxiety

   C. Indifference

   D. Hyperactivity

2. Which therapy is particularly effective for managing stress and emotional distress in COPD patients?

   A. Antibiotic therapy

   B. Cognitive-behavioral therapy (CBT)

   C. Chemotherapy

   D. Antiviral therapy

3. What type of support group is beneficial for COPD patients?

A. Weight loss support groups

B. COPD support groups

C. Financial advice groups

D. Professional networking groups

4. Regular physical activity for COPD patients can help improve which of the following?

A. Lung function directly

B. Mental health

C. Bone density only

D. Vision clarity

5. Why are family and friends considered an important support system for COPD patients?

A. They can prescribe medications.

B. They offer emotional support and help manage daily tasks.

C. They provide professional counseling.

D. They can perform surgical procedures.

6. Depression and anxiety in COPD patients can lead to:

A. Improved medication adherence

B. Fewer hospitalizations

C. Reduced adherence to treatment plans

D. Increased lung capacity

7. Which of the following is NOT a goal of pulmonary rehabilitation counseling?

A. To cure COPD

B. To teach stress management techniques

C. To provide strategies for managing breathlessness

D. To promote lifestyle modifications

8. The integration of which service into COPD care can help address psychological impacts of the disease?

A. Legal services

B. Cosmetic surgery

C. Counseling services

D. Financial planning

9. How does participation in support groups benefit COPD patients?

A. It directly increases oxygen levels.

B. It offers a platform for sharing experiences and coping strategies.

C. It eliminates the need for medication.

D. It provides a cure for COPD.

10. Effective coping strategies for managing COPD include all EXCEPT:

    A. Ignoring symptoms to avoid stress

    B. Seeking professional help for mental health issues

    C. Engaging in regular physical activity within individual limits

    D. Educating oneself and others about COPD

Answers:

1. B. Anxiety

2. B. Cognitive-behavioral therapy (CBT)

3. B. COPD support groups

4. B. Mental health

5. B. They offer emotional support and help manage daily tasks.

6. C. Reduced adherence to treatment plans

7. A. To cure COPD

8. C. Counseling services

9. B. It offers a platform for sharing experiences and coping strategies.

10. A. Ignoring symptoms to avoid stress

Chapter 10: COPD and Comorbid Conditions

10.1 Heart Disease and COPD: A Dangerous Duo

The Interconnection Between Heart Disease and COPD

Chronic Obstructive Pulmonary Disease (COPD) and heart disease often coexist, creating a complex health challenge for patients. The overlap is not coincidental; the two conditions share common risk factors and pathophysiological mechanisms that can exacerbate each other, significantly impacting patient outcomes and quality of life.

Shared Risk Factors

- **Smoking:** The leading cause of both COPD and many forms of heart disease, smoking damages the lungs and the cardiovascular system.

- **Age:** The risk of developing both conditions increases with age due to the cumulative effects of exposure to risk factors and the natural aging process of the heart and lungs.

- **Inactivity:** Physical inactivity is a risk factor for the progression of COPD and the development of heart disease, as it contributes to declining lung function and poor cardiovascular health.

Pathophysiological Links

- **Systemic Inflammation:** COPD is characterized by chronic inflammation, which can also contribute to the development of atherosclerosis, a key factor in heart disease.

- **Oxygen Deprivation:** Impaired gas exchange in COPD can lead to decreased oxygen levels in the blood, forcing the heart to work harder to deliver oxygen to the body, which can exacerbate existing heart conditions or even lead to new ones.

- **Pulmonary Hypertension:** COPD can cause increased blood pressure in the arteries of the lungs (pulmonary hypertension), placing additional strain on the right side of the heart.

Impact on Management and Treatment

The coexistence of heart disease and COPD necessitates a careful, coordinated approach to management:

- **Integrated Care Plans:** Treatment plans should address both conditions simultaneously, optimizing medications to avoid potential conflicts and side effects.

- **Monitoring and Adjustment:** Regular monitoring of both cardiac and pulmonary functions is essential, with adjustments to treatment plans as needed based on changes in either condition.

- **Lifestyle Modifications:** Smoking cessation, increased physical activity, and dietary changes are critical components of managing both conditions.

- **Patient Education:** Understanding the link between heart disease and COPD is vital for patients to recognize the importance of comprehensive management strategies.

Conclusion

Heart disease and COPD form a dangerous duo that requires comprehensive and integrated management strategies to mitigate the risks and complications associated with their coexistence. Recognizing the shared risk factors and intertwined pathophysiology allows healthcare providers to develop effective treatment plans that address the complexity of having both conditions, ultimately improving patient outcomes and quality of life.

10.2 The Interplay Between COPD and Diabetes

Understanding the Relationship

The relationship between Chronic Obstructive Pulmonary Disease (COPD) and diabetes mellitus is complex and bidirectional. Both diseases share common risk factors and can influence each other's progression and management. The presence of diabetes can affect the severity of COPD, while COPD may increase the risk of developing type 2 diabetes due to systemic inflammation and steroid use.

Shared Risk Factors

- **Smoking:** A major risk factor for both COPD and type 2 diabetes, smoking can lead to insulin resistance and impaired lung function.

- **Obesity:** Increases the risk of type 2 diabetes and can worsen COPD outcomes due to increased inflammation and decreased lung function.

- **Physical Inactivity:** Contributes to the development of both conditions by promoting insulin resistance and weakening respiratory muscles.

Impact of Diabetes on COPD

Diabetes can complicate the management of COPD in several ways:

- **Worsened Lung Function:** High blood sugar levels can lead to inflammation and damage in lung tissues, exacerbating respiratory symptoms.

- **Increased Risk of Infections:** Diabetes can impair the immune system, making individuals more susceptible to respiratory infections, which can trigger COPD exacerbations.

- **Medication Interactions:** Some medications used to treat COPD, especially systemic corticosteroids, can increase blood sugar levels, complicating diabetes management.

Impact of COPD on Diabetes

- **Increased Insulin Resistance:** The systemic inflammation associated with COPD can contribute to the development of insulin resistance, a precursor to type 2 diabetes.

- **Medication Side Effects:** Corticosteroids, commonly used during COPD exacerbations, can elevate blood glucose levels, requiring adjustments in diabetes management.

Strategies for Managing COPD and Diabetes Together

- **Integrated Care Approach:** Healthcare providers should address both conditions simultaneously, monitoring lung function and blood glucose levels regularly.

- **Lifestyle Modifications:** Quitting smoking, adopting a healthy diet, and increasing physical activity can significantly impact the management of both COPD and diabetes.

- **Medication Management:** Careful selection of medications to avoid exacerbating either condition, and adjusting dosages as necessary based on the patient's overall health status.

- **Patient Education:** Educating patients about the interplay between COPD and diabetes, including the importance of medication adherence, lifestyle changes, and regular monitoring.

Conclusion

The interplay between COPD and diabetes underscores the need for a coordinated, multidisciplinary approach to patient care. Recognizing and managing the bidirectional influences of these chronic conditions can help improve patient outcomes, reduce exacerbations, and enhance quality of life. Lifestyle modifications, integrated care plans, and patient education are key components of effective management strategies for individuals affected by both COPD and diabetes.

10.3 Osteoporosis and COPD: Addressing Bone Health

The Link Between COPD and Osteoporosis

Osteoporosis, a condition characterized by weakened bones and increased fracture risk, is notably more prevalent in individuals with Chronic Obstructive Pulmonary Disease (COPD). The connection between these two conditions is multifaceted, involving shared risk factors, the effects of chronic inflammation, and the impact of COPD treatments on bone health.

Why COPD Patients Are at Increased Risk

- **Systemic Inflammation:** COPD is associated with chronic systemic inflammation, which can lead to increased bone resorption and decreased bone formation, contributing to osteoporosis.

- **Corticosteroid Use:** Long-term use of systemic corticosteroids, a common treatment for COPD exacerbations, can decrease bone density and increase the risk of osteoporosis.

- **Physical Inactivity:** The limitations on physical activity often experienced by individuals with COPD can lead to decreased bone strength and mass.

- **Nutritional Deficiencies:** COPD patients may have deficiencies in essential nutrients for bone health, such as vitamin D and calcium, due to dietary restrictions or malabsorption.

Strategies for Addressing Bone Health in COPD

- **Bone Density Screening:** Regular screening for osteoporosis should be part of the management plan for patients with COPD, especially those with risk factors for bone loss.

- **Optimizing Nutritional Intake:** Ensuring adequate intake of calcium and vitamin D, either through diet or supplements, is crucial for maintaining bone health.

- **Exercise and Rehabilitation:** Weight-bearing and resistance exercises, as part of a pulmonary rehabilitation program, can help improve bone density and muscle strength.

- **Smoking Cessation:** Quitting smoking can slow the progression of both COPD and osteoporosis, as smoking is a risk factor for both conditions.

- **Medication Management:** For patients requiring long-term corticosteroid therapy, the use of the lowest effective dose and consideration of alternative treatments can help minimize the risk of osteoporosis. Additionally, medications specifically designed to treat osteoporosis, such as bisphosphonates, may be recommended.

Monitoring and Intervention

- **Regular Monitoring:** Alongside COPD management, monitoring for signs of osteoporosis and initiating treatment early can prevent fractures and improve quality of life.

- **Fall Prevention:** Implementing measures to reduce the risk of falls, a common cause of fractures in individuals with osteoporosis, is important. This can include home modifications, balance exercises, and reviewing medications that may affect balance.

Conclusion

The relationship between COPD and osteoporosis highlights the importance of a comprehensive approach to patient care that addresses not only pulmonary health but also bone health. By integrating strategies for managing osteoporosis into the care plan for COPD patients, healthcare providers can help mitigate the impact of both conditions, improve patient outcomes, and enhance quality of life.

10.4 Exercise: 10 MCQs with Answers at the End

Test your knowledge on COPD and its comorbid conditions, including heart disease, diabetes, osteoporosis, and their management strategies, with these multiple-choice questions. Answers are provided at the end for self-assessment.

1. What is a common comorbidity of COPD that affects bone health?

   A. Osteoporosis

   B. Hypertension

   C. Diabetes mellitus

   D. Hyperlipidemia

2. Which medication used in COPD management can contribute to the risk of developing osteoporosis?

   A. Antibiotics

   B. Short-acting bronchodilators

   C. Systemic corticosteroids

   D. Antihistamines

3. How does physical inactivity related to COPD contribute to osteoporosis?

A. By increasing bone density

B. By reducing calcium absorption

C. By decreasing bone mass and strength

D. By improving vitamin D synthesis

4. Which lifestyle modification can benefit both COPD and heart disease management?

A. Smoking cessation

B. Increased salt intake

C. Sedentary lifestyle

D. High-fat diet

5. Regular screening for which condition should be part of COPD management due to its increased prevalence?

A. Osteoporosis

B. Migraine

C. Epilepsy

D. Psoriasis

6. How does systemic inflammation in COPD patients contribute to heart disease?

A. By lowering cholesterol levels

B. By improving heart rate variability

C. By promoting atherosclerosis

D. By decreasing blood pressure

7. Vitamin D supplementation is important in COPD patients for managing:

A. High blood sugar levels

B. Bone health

C. Lung infections

D. Blood clotting

8. Which exercise type is beneficial for improving bone health in COPD patients?

A. Weight-bearing exercises

B. Breathing exercises only

C. Stretching exercises

D. Relaxation exercises

9. The risk of which condition is increased in COPD patients due to corticosteroid use and chronic inflammation?

A. Osteoporosis

B. Hypothyroidism

C. Gastroesophageal reflux disease (GERD)

D. Acne

10. Management of COPD and diabetes together includes:

A. Ignoring blood sugar levels when prescribing steroids

B. Encouraging a high-carbohydrate diet

C. Monitoring and adjusting treatment plans as needed

D. Avoiding physical activity to reduce hypoglycemia risk

Answers:

1. A. Osteoporosis

2. C. Systemic corticosteroids

3. C. By decreasing bone mass and strength

4. A. Smoking cessation

5. A. Osteoporosis

6. C. By promoting atherosclerosis

7. B. Bone health

8. A. Weight-bearing exercises

9. A. Osteoporosis

10. C. Monitoring and adjusting treatment plans as needed

Chapter 11: The Future of COPD Treatment

11.1 Emerging Therapies and Clinical Trials

Innovations in COPD Management

The landscape of Chronic Obstructive Pulmonary Disease (COPD) treatment is evolving, with ongoing research aimed at developing new therapies to better manage the disease, improve patient outcomes, and potentially alter its course. Emerging therapies and clinical trials focus on targeting the underlying mechanisms of COPD, reducing exacerbations, and improving lung function and quality of life.

Areas of Research and Emerging Therapies

- **Anti-inflammatory Agents:** New classes of anti-inflammatory medications are being developed to more effectively reduce the chronic inflammation associated with COPD. These include inhibitors of specific cytokines and pathways implicated in the inflammatory process.

- **Bronchodilators:** Research continues into novel bronchodilators with longer durations of action and improved efficacy, aiming to enhance symptom control and reduce the burden of treatment.

- **Gene Therapy:** Early-stage research is exploring the potential of gene therapy to correct genetic defects associated with COPD or to introduce genes that can reduce inflammation and repair lung tissue.

- **Regenerative Medicine:** Stem cell therapy and tissue engineering hold promise for regenerating damaged lung tissue. Clinical trials are investigating the safety and efficacy of stem cell therapies in repairing the alveoli and improving lung function in COPD patients.

- **Biologic Therapies:** Targeted biologic therapies, such as monoclonal antibodies, are being tested for their ability to target specific molecules and pathways involved in COPD pathogenesis, particularly for patients with severe disease and frequent exacerbations.

- **Vaccines:** Research is ongoing into vaccines that could prevent the onset of COPD in high-risk individuals or reduce the frequency of viral and bacterial exacerbations in patients with established disease.

Challenges and Considerations

- **Personalized Medicine:** As understanding of the molecular and genetic basis of COPD improves, there is an increasing focus on personalized medicine — tailoring treatments to the specific characteristics of an individual's disease to optimize outcomes.

- **Clinical Trials:** Participation in clinical trials is critical for the development of new therapies. These studies must carefully balance efficacy and safety, and patients should be fully informed of potential risks and benefits.

- **Access and Cost:** Emerging therapies, particularly those involving advanced technology or biologic agents, can be costly. Ensuring access to these treatments for all patients who could benefit remains a challenge.

Conclusion

The future of COPD treatment is bright, with numerous promising therapies on the horizon. Ongoing research and clinical trials are essential for bringing these innovations from the laboratory to the clinic, offering hope for improved management and potentially transformative outcomes for individuals living with COPD. As these new treatments emerge, it will be important to integrate them into comprehensive care strategies, considering the individual needs and preferences of each patient.

11.2 Gene Therapy and Regenerative Medicine

Revolutionizing COPD Treatment

The fields of gene therapy and regenerative medicine represent the cutting edge of research into treatments for Chronic Obstructive Pulmonary Disease (COPD). These innovative approaches aim not only to alleviate symptoms but also to address the underlying causes of the disease, offering the potential for more durable and transformative outcomes.

Gene Therapy: A New Horizon

Gene therapy involves the delivery of specific genes into a patient's cells to treat or prevent disease. In COPD, this approach could correct genetic defects associated with the disease or introduce new genes to help repair damaged lung tissue or reduce inflammation.

- **Targeting Genetic Factors:** For patients with alpha-1 antitrypsin deficiency, a genetic condition associated with emphysema, gene therapy could potentially deliver a functional copy of the alpha-1 antitrypsin gene to the lungs.

- **Anti-inflammatory Genes:** Introducing genes that encode anti-inflammatory proteins could help to reduce the chronic inflammation that characterizes COPD.

- **Challenges and Future Directions:** Gene therapy for COPD is still in the early stages of research, with challenges related to the efficient and safe delivery of genes to lung tissues. Ongoing studies aim to overcome these hurdles and move closer to clinical applications.

Regenerative Medicine: Restoring Lung Function

Regenerative medicine seeks to repair or replace damaged tissues and organs. In the context of COPD, this could involve stimulating the regeneration of lung tissue or using stem cells to repair the alveoli and airways.

- **Stem Cell Therapy:** Early clinical trials are exploring the use of stem cells, derived from bone marrow or other sources, to regenerate damaged lung tissue. These cells have the potential to reduce inflammation, promote healing, and restore lung function.

- **Tissue Engineering:** This approach involves creating lung tissue in the lab that can be transplanted into patients. While still experimental, it offers the possibility of replacing diseased lung tissue with healthy tissue.

- **Current Status and Considerations:** While promising, regenerative medicine for COPD faces challenges, including understanding the best sources of stem cells, ensuring the safety of these therapies, and achieving durable integration and function of regenerated tissues.

Conclusion

Gene therapy and regenerative medicine hold great promise for the future of COPD treatment, with the potential to fundamentally change the way the disease is managed. By targeting the genetic and cellular foundations of COPD, these approaches aim to repair lung damage, reduce inflammation, and improve lung function. Although still in the research phase, the ongoing development of these therapies offers hope for more effective and restorative treatments for COPD in the future.

11.3 Personalized Medicine: Tailoring Treatment to the Individual

The Evolution of COPD Treatment

Personalized medicine represents a paradigm shift in the treatment of Chronic Obstructive Pulmonary Disease (COPD), moving away from a one-size-fits-all approach to care that is specifically tailored to the unique genetic makeup, lifestyle, and disease characteristics of each individual. This approach seeks to optimize treatment efficacy, minimize side effects, and improve overall patient outcomes.

Components of Personalized Medicine in COPD

- **Genetic Profiling:** Identifying genetic factors that influence COPD risk, progression, and response to treatment can help in developing targeted therapies. For instance, patients with alpha-1 antitrypsin deficiency may benefit from specific replacement therapies.

- **Biomarkers:** Biomarkers are measurable indicators of disease state or treatment response. In COPD, biomarkers can help in diagnosing the disease, predicting exacerbations, and monitoring response to treatment, guiding the customization of therapy.

- **Pharmacogenomics:** This field studies how genes affect a person's response to drugs. In COPD, pharmacogenomic testing can identify which medications are likely to be most effective or pose risks of side effects for individual patients.

Benefits of Personalized Medicine

- **Enhanced Treatment Efficacy:** By tailoring treatments to the individual's specific disease characteristics and genetic profile, personalized medicine can significantly improve the efficacy of COPD management.

- **Reduced Adverse Effects:** Personalized medicine can help avoid medications that are likely to cause adverse effects in certain individuals, improving patient safety and comfort.

- **Improved Disease Management:** Personalized approaches can lead to better disease control, fewer hospitalizations, and an improved quality of life for COPD patients.

Challenges and Future Directions

- **Data Integration:** The success of personalized medicine depends on the integration of complex data sets, including genetic information, biomarkers, and clinical data, requiring sophisticated analytical tools and interdisciplinary collaboration.

- **Accessibility:** Ensuring that personalized medicine approaches are accessible to all patients, regardless of socioeconomic status or geographic location, is a significant challenge.

- **Ethical Considerations:** The use of genetic information and biomarkers raises ethical questions regarding privacy, consent, and the potential for discrimination.

Conclusion

Personalized medicine in COPD has the potential to transform the management of the disease, offering treatments that are specifically designed to match the individual characteristics of each patient. While challenges remain in implementing personalized medicine widely, ongoing research and advances in genomics and data analysis are paving the way for more precise, effective, and patient-centered approaches to COPD care.

11.4 Exercise: 10 MCQs with Answers at the End

Test your knowledge on the future of COPD treatment, including emerging therapies, gene therapy, regenerative medicine, and personalized medicine, with these multiple-choice questions. Answers are provided at the end for self-assessment.

1. What is the goal of gene therapy in COPD treatment?

   A. To increase physical strength

   B. To correct genetic defects or introduce beneficial genes

   C. To replace traditional medications

   D. To enhance lung capacity instantly

2. Which area of research focuses on using stem cells to repair damaged lung tissue in COPD?

   A. Pharmacogenomics

   B. Regenerative medicine

C. Biomarker identification

D. Genetic profiling

3. Personalized medicine in COPD is characterized by:

A. A standardized treatment for all patients

B. Treatments tailored to individual genetic makeup and disease characteristics

C. Avoiding the use of modern medications

D. Sole reliance on physical therapy

4. Emerging therapies in COPD aim to:

A. Temporarily relieve symptoms

B. Address the underlying mechanisms of the disease

C. Focus solely on lifestyle changes

D. Eliminate the need for patient participation

5. What challenge is associated with implementing gene therapy in COPD?

A. Immediate risk of lung damage

B. Efficient and safe delivery of genes to lung tissues

C. Excessive cost savings

D. Reducing physical activity levels

6. Regenerative medicine in COPD might include:

   A. Daily use of corticosteroids

   B. Tissue engineering and stem cell therapy

   C. Elimination of all medications

   D. Strict dietary restrictions

7. The use of biomarkers in COPD treatment can help with:

   A. Predicting weather changes

   B. Diagnosing the disease and monitoring treatment response

   C. Increasing dependency on oxygen therapy

   D. Decreasing the need for patient education

8. One of the benefits of personalized medicine for COPD patients is:

   A. Reduced adverse effects from treatments

   B. Increased need for hospitalization

   C. Uniform treatment protocols for all patients

   D. Discouragement of exercise and rehabilitation

9. Which of the following is NOT a focus of current COPD research?

   A. Developing vaccines to prevent COPD

   B. Finding ways to reduce physical exercise

C. Identifying new anti-inflammatory agents

D. Exploring the efficacy of biologic therapies

10. Pharmacogenomics in COPD treatment helps to:

A. Increase the effectiveness of physical therapy

B. Identify which medications are likely to be most effective for an individual

C. Replace all other forms of COPD treatment

D. Promote a one-size-fits-all approach to medication

Answers:

1. B. To correct genetic defects or introduce beneficial genes

2. B. Regenerative medicine

3. B. Treatments tailored to individual genetic makeup and disease characteristics

4. B. Address the underlying mechanisms of the disease

5. B. Efficient and safe delivery of genes to lung tissues

6. B. Tissue engineering and stem cell therapy

7. B. Diagnosing the disease and monitoring treatment response

8. A. Reduced adverse effects from treatments

9. B. Finding ways to reduce physical exercise

10. B. Identify which medications are likely to be most effective for an individual

Chapter 12: Global Perspectives on COPD

12.1 Epidemiology: A Worldwide Overview

Understanding COPD on a Global Scale

Chronic Obstructive Pulmonary Disease (COPD) is a major cause of morbidity and mortality worldwide, presenting significant challenges to public health systems across different countries. The global epidemiology of COPD reveals diverse patterns and trends, influenced by factors such as smoking rates, air pollution, occupational exposures, and access to healthcare.

Global Prevalence and Trends

- COPD affects millions of people around the globe, with estimates suggesting that it may be the third leading cause of death worldwide.

- Prevalence rates vary significantly between countries and regions, influenced by differences in smoking habits, environmental factors, and diagnostic practices.

- While traditionally considered a disease of older adults, COPD is increasingly diagnosed in younger populations, partly due to better awareness and diagnostic capabilities.

Risk Factors

- **Tobacco Smoke:** The primary risk factor for COPD globally, including both direct smoking and exposure to secondhand smoke.

- **Air Pollution:** Both outdoor and indoor air pollution contribute to the burden of COPD, with indoor pollution from biomass fuel use being a significant issue in developing countries.

- **Occupational Exposures:** Exposure to dust, chemicals, and fumes in certain workplaces increases the risk of developing COPD.

- **Genetic Factors:** Variations in genetic susceptibility to COPD are observed, with alpha-1 antitrypsin deficiency being a well-known genetic risk factor.

Challenges in COPD Management Worldwide

- **Diagnosis and Awareness:** Underdiagnosis of COPD remains a significant challenge in many countries, partly due to limited awareness and access to diagnostic tools like spirometry.

- **Access to Care:** Variability in access to healthcare services and COPD treatments exists between and within countries, influenced by economic and healthcare system factors.

- **Cultural and Socioeconomic Factors:** Cultural beliefs, healthcare-seeking behavior, and socioeconomic status can influence COPD management and outcomes.

Global Initiatives and Collaborations

- Several international initiatives aim to improve COPD awareness, prevention, and management, including the Global Initiative for Chronic Obstructive Lung Disease (GOLD) and the World Health Organization's (WHO) efforts to reduce tobacco use and improve air quality.

- Collaborative research efforts are underway to better understand the genetic and environmental factors contributing to COPD and to develop more effective treatments.

Conclusion

COPD is a global health issue that requires a coordinated international response to improve prevention, diagnosis, and management. Addressing the challenges of COPD on a global scale will necessitate multifaceted strategies, encompassing public health interventions, improved access to care, and ongoing research to understand and mitigate the impact of this chronic disease.

12.2 Healthcare Systems and Access to Care

Navigating COPD Care Across Different Healthcare Systems

The management of Chronic Obstructive Pulmonary Disease (COPD) can vary significantly across different healthcare systems around the world. Access to care, the availability of treatments, and the approach to managing COPD are influenced by the structure and resources of each country's healthcare system.

Variability in Healthcare Systems

- **Universal Healthcare Systems:** Countries with universal healthcare systems typically offer a wide range of COPD management services at little or no direct cost to the patient. However, there may be challenges related to wait times for certain services or limitations in the availability of the latest treatments.

- **Private Healthcare Systems:** In countries with predominantly private healthcare systems, access to COPD care may depend on one's ability to pay or the quality of their health insurance coverage. While access to cutting-edge treatments may be quicker, the cost can be a significant barrier for many.

- **Mixed Healthcare Systems:** Many countries operate mixed healthcare systems, offering both public and private options. The quality and accessibility of COPD care can vary widely within these systems, often depending on personal or socioeconomic factors.

Challenges in Access to COPD Care

- **Diagnosis:** Early diagnosis of COPD is crucial for effective management but remains a challenge in many parts of the world due to a lack of awareness and limited access to diagnostic tools like spirometry.

- **Treatment:** Access to a full range of pharmacological treatments, pulmonary rehabilitation, and oxygen therapy can be limited by geographical location, healthcare infrastructure, and economic factors.

- **Education and Support:** Patient education and support services, critical for effective disease management, may not be widely available in all healthcare systems, particularly in resource-limited settings.

Strategies to Improve Access

- **Strengthening Primary Care:** Enhancing the capabilities of primary care services to diagnose and manage COPD can improve access to care and reduce the need for hospitalizations.

- **Leveraging Technology:** Telemedicine and digital health tools can extend the reach of COPD care, offering remote monitoring and support, especially in underserved areas.

- **International Collaboration:** Global health initiatives and partnerships can help to build capacity, share best practices, and distribute resources more evenly across countries.

- **Patient Advocacy:** Advocacy groups play a crucial role in raising awareness about COPD, advocating for better access to care, and supporting research into new treatments.

Conclusion

Access to comprehensive COPD care varies significantly across different healthcare systems, with disparities in diagnosis, treatment, and support services. Efforts to improve access to care require a multifaceted approach, including strengthening primary care, leveraging technology, fostering international collaboration, and advocating for patients' needs. Addressing these challenges is essential to improving outcomes for individuals living with COPD worldwide.

12.3 Cultural Influences on Treatment and Management

The Role of Culture in COPD Care

Cultural beliefs and practices can significantly influence how Chronic Obstructive Pulmonary Disease (COPD) is treated and managed. These cultural factors can affect patients' perceptions of illness, their approach to seeking medical care, adherence to treatment plans, and engagement in lifestyle modifications recommended for managing COPD.

Understanding Cultural Influences

- **Perceptions of Illness:** Cultural beliefs can shape how symptoms are interpreted and when medical help is sought. In some cultures, respiratory symptoms might be considered a normal part of aging or attributed to factors outside of medical control, delaying diagnosis and treatment.

- **Attitudes Towards Healthcare:** Trust in medical professionals and willingness to engage with healthcare systems can vary, influenced by past experiences, societal beliefs, and healthcare accessibility. This can impact the effectiveness of COPD management strategies.

- **Use of Traditional Remedies:** Many cultures have traditional remedies or practices for health issues, including respiratory conditions. While some may offer symptomatic relief, reliance on these methods alone can hinder effective COPD management.

- **Smoking and Tobacco Use:** Cultural norms surrounding smoking and tobacco use play a significant role in COPD risk. Social acceptability, gender roles, and religious beliefs can influence smoking behaviors, affecting the prevalence and management of COPD.

- **Dietary Practices:** Nutritional habits and preferences, often rooted in culture, can impact COPD management. Diets rich in anti-inflammatory foods may support lung health, while other dietary patterns could exacerbate symptoms.

Strategies for Culturally Sensitive COPD Care

- **Cultural Competence in Healthcare Providers:** Training in cultural competence can help healthcare providers understand and respect cultural differences, improving patient communication and trust.

- **Incorporating Traditional Practices:** Where appropriate, integrating traditional remedies or practices into COPD management plans can enhance patient adherence and respect cultural values.

- **Tailored Patient Education:** Educational materials and interventions should be culturally sensitive and available in multiple languages to ensure they are accessible and relevant to diverse patient populations.

- **Community Engagement:** Involving community leaders and using peer support groups can facilitate culturally relevant health education and encourage engagement with COPD management strategies.

Conclusion

Cultural influences play a critical role in the treatment and management of COPD, affecting everything from the perception of symptoms to adherence to treatment plans. Recognizing and addressing these cultural factors is essential for providing effective, personalized COPD care. Culturally sensitive approaches, including education, communication, and the integration of cultural practices, can improve outcomes for COPD patients across diverse communities.

12.4 Exercise: 10 MCQs with Answers at the End

Test your knowledge on the global perspectives of COPD, including epidemiology, healthcare systems, cultural influences, and strategies for improving worldwide COPD care, with these multiple-choice questions. Answers are provided at the end for self-assessment.

1. COPD is projected to be the third leading cause of death worldwide due to factors like:

   A. Increased physical activity

   B. Smoking and air pollution

   C. Improved healthcare access

   D. Decreased use of biomass fuels

2. A significant barrier to COPD care in developing countries is:

A. Overdiagnosis

B. Lack of awareness and diagnostic tools

C. Excessive reliance on traditional medicine

D. Too much emphasis on preventive care

3. Cultural beliefs can impact COPD management by influencing:

A. Global warming trends

B. Perceptions of illness and healthcare utilization

C. The development of new COPD medications

D. International travel regulations

4. The use of traditional remedies for COPD:

A. Is universally effective across all cultures

B. Can sometimes complement conventional treatments

C. Always leads to improved lung function

D. Is recommended as the sole treatment method

5. In countries with universal healthcare systems, a challenge for COPD patients might be:

A. Immediate access to all types of treatment

B. Long wait times for certain services

C. Lack of any form of healthcare coverage

D. Excessive costs for pulmonary rehabilitation

6. Strategies to improve global COPD care include:

A. Reducing physical activity to conserve energy

B. Strengthening primary care and leveraging technology

C. Ignoring cultural influences on health behaviors

D. Focusing solely on pharmacological treatments

7. Pharmacogenomics in COPD treatment can help:

A. Predict weather changes affecting symptoms

B. Identify medications likely to be effective for individual patients

C. Eliminate the need for oxygen therapy

D. Increase dependency on inhaled corticosteroids

8. Cultural competence in healthcare providers is important for:

A. Discouraging the use of traditional remedies

B. Ensuring treatments align with cultural beliefs and practices

C. Implementing a one-size-fits-all approach to COPD care

D. Promoting smoking in cultural contexts where it is prevalent

9. An emerging area of COPD research focuses on:

A. Developing vaccines to prevent exacerbations

B. Encouraging smoking as a stress-relief method

C. Phasing out the use of bronchodilators

D. Eliminating the need for spirometry in diagnosis

10. Access to COPD care in private healthcare systems is primarily influenced by:

A. The patient's ability to pay or quality of health insurance

B. The availability of natural remedies

C. Universal access to all treatments

D. Government-imposed healthcare regulations

Answers:

1. B. Smoking and air pollution

2. B. Lack of awareness and diagnostic tools

3. B. Perceptions of illness and healthcare utilization

4. B. Can sometimes complement conventional treatments

5. B. Long wait times for certain services

6. B. Strengthening primary care and leveraging technology

7. B. Identify medications likely to be effective for individual patients

8. B. Ensuring treatments align with cultural beliefs and practices

9. A. Developing vaccines to prevent exacerbations

10. A. The patient's ability to pay or quality of health insurance

Chapter 13: Environmental and Occupational Risks

13.1 Air Quality and Pollution: Impact on Lung Health

The Perilous Effects of Poor Air Quality

Air quality, particularly the presence of pollutants in the atmosphere, plays a significant role in lung health and the development and exacerbation of respiratory diseases such as Chronic Obstructive Pulmonary Disease (COPD). Both outdoor and indoor air pollution are recognized as major environmental risk factors that can have detrimental effects on the respiratory system.

Sources and Types of Air Pollution

- **Outdoor Pollution:** Comes from various sources including industrial emissions, vehicle exhaust, wildfires, and agricultural practices. Common pollutants include particulate matter (PM), nitrogen dioxide (NO2), sulfur dioxide (SO2), and ozone (O3).

- **Indoor Pollution:** Arises from the use of biomass fuels for cooking and heating, tobacco smoke, building materials, and household cleaning products. Indoor air can be contaminated with pollutants like carbon monoxide (CO), particulate matter, and volatile organic compounds (VOCs).

Impact on Lung Health

- **Inflammation and Oxidative Stress:** Exposure to air pollutants can cause inflammation and oxidative stress in the respiratory tract, leading to damage of lung tissues.

- **Exacerbation of COPD:** Pollutants can irritate the airways, leading to increased COPD symptoms, such as coughing, wheezing, and breathlessness, and can trigger exacerbations.

- **Increased Risk of Respiratory Infections:** Polluted air can impair the lung's defense mechanisms, making it easier for infections to take hold, which can further compromise lung function in individuals with COPD.

- **Long-Term Lung Function Decline:** Chronic exposure to high levels of pollution can accelerate the decline in lung function and contribute to the development of COPD or worsen existing disease.

Strategies to Mitigate the Impact

- **Reducing Exposure:** On days when air quality is poor, individuals, especially those with pre-existing lung conditions, should stay indoors as much as possible and use air purifiers to reduce indoor pollution levels.

- **Public Health Policies:** Implementing and enforcing regulations to reduce emissions from vehicles and industries can significantly improve outdoor air quality.

- **Personal Protective Measures:** Wearing masks designed to filter out pollutants and ensuring good ventilation when using indoor sources of combustion can help reduce exposure.

- **Promoting Clean Energy:** Transitioning to clean energy sources for cooking, heating, and power generation can decrease indoor and outdoor air pollution.

Conclusion

The link between air quality, pollution, and lung health is unequivocal, with significant implications for the development and management of COPD. Addressing air pollution requires concerted efforts at both individual and policy levels to mitigate its impact on respiratory health and reduce the burden of lung diseases globally.

13.2 Workplace Hazards and Protective Strategies

Occupational Risks for Lung Health

Workplace environments can expose individuals to various hazards that pose significant risks to lung health, including the development and exacerbation of Chronic Obstructive Pulmonary Disease (COPD). Recognizing and mitigating these occupational risks are crucial steps in preventing occupational lung diseases.

Common Workplace Hazards

- **Dusts:** Fine particulate matter from construction materials, textiles, or agricultural products can cause respiratory problems.

- **Chemicals:** Exposure to certain gases, vapors, and fumes from chemicals used in manufacturing, painting, or cleaning can damage the lungs.

- **Smoke and Combustion Products:** Firefighters and workers in environments with open flames or combustion engines are at risk from smoke inhalation.

- **Biological Agents:** Exposure to molds, animal dander, or other biological agents in settings like healthcare, agriculture, or waste management can trigger or worsen respiratory conditions.

Impact on COPD

Occupational exposures can lead to the development of COPD or worsen existing conditions by causing airway inflammation, reducing lung function, and increasing the frequency of respiratory symptoms and exacerbations.

Protective Strategies

- **Risk Assessment and Monitoring:** Identifying and assessing respiratory hazards in the workplace is the first step in protecting workers. Regular monitoring can help manage known risks and identify new ones.

- **Use of Personal Protective Equipment (PPE):** Respirators, masks, and other protective gear can significantly reduce exposure to harmful agents. Proper fit and compliance with usage guidelines are essential for effectiveness.

- **Ventilation and Air Quality Control:** Enhancing ventilation systems and using air cleaning technologies can lower the concentration of airborne pollutants in the workplace.

- **Training and Education:** Workers should be educated about the risks associated with their jobs and trained in the use of protective measures and equipment.

- **Health Surveillance:** Regular health checks for workers in high-risk occupations can help detect early signs of respiratory conditions, allowing for timely intervention and management.

- **Regulatory Compliance:** Adhering to occupational health and safety regulations and guidelines is crucial for minimizing workplace hazards and protecting workers' health.

Conclusion

Occupational hazards are a significant concern for lung health and the management of COPD. Implementing comprehensive protective strategies, including the use of PPE, improving workplace conditions, and ensuring regulatory compliance, can help mitigate these risks. Continued efforts to educate workers and employers about the importance of respiratory health and safety are vital for preventing occupational lung diseases.

13.3 Climate Change and Respiratory Health

Climate Change: A Growing Threat to Lung Health

Climate change is increasingly recognized as a critical public health issue, with profound implications for respiratory health. Rising temperatures, changes in weather patterns, and increased frequency of wildfires and air pollution events all contribute to worsening lung health and exacerbating conditions like Chronic Obstructive Pulmonary Disease (COPD).

Impact of Climate Change on Respiratory Health

- **Increased Air Pollution:** Climate change contributes to higher concentrations of ground-level ozone and particulate matter, both of which can aggravate COPD symptoms and lead to exacerbations.

- **Wildfires:** Increased frequency and intensity of wildfires, driven by hotter, drier conditions, produce smoke and airborne particulates that can significantly impair lung function and exacerbate respiratory diseases.

- **Allergens:** Rising temperatures and carbon dioxide levels lead to longer pollen seasons and higher pollen concentrations, worsening allergic reactions and respiratory symptoms in sensitive individuals.

- **Heatwaves:** Extreme heat can directly stress the respiratory system and exacerbate lung conditions, particularly in individuals with pre-existing COPD.

- **Infectious Diseases:** Changes in climate patterns can affect the distribution and transmission of respiratory infections, potentially leading to more frequent and severe infections.

Strategies for Mitigating the Impact

- **Public Awareness and Education:** Raising awareness about the link between climate change and respiratory health is essential for motivating action and preparedness.

- **Reducing Exposure:** During periods of poor air quality, such as wildfire smoke events or heatwaves, individuals with COPD should stay indoors with air conditioning and air purifiers to reduce exposure to pollutants and heat.

- **Policy and Advocacy:** Advocating for policies that address the root causes of climate change, reduce emissions, and promote cleaner air can help mitigate the impact on respiratory health.

- **Healthcare Preparedness:** Healthcare systems need to be prepared for increased demand during environmental events that affect air quality, with plans in place for managing exacerbations and supporting vulnerable populations.

- **Research and Monitoring:** Ongoing research is needed to better understand the specific impacts of climate change on respiratory diseases and to develop effective strategies for prevention and management.

Conclusion

The effects of climate change on respiratory health are significant and multifaceted, posing challenges for individuals with COPD and other lung conditions. By understanding these impacts and implementing strategies to reduce exposure and advocate for cleaner air, it is possible to mitigate some of the adverse effects of climate change on lung health. Collaboration between public health officials, healthcare providers, policymakers, and communities is essential for addressing this global health threat.

13.4 Exercise: 10 MCQs with Answers at the End

Evaluate your understanding of environmental and occupational risks related to COPD, including air quality and pollution, workplace hazards, and the effects of climate change on respiratory health, with these multiple-choice questions. Answers are provided at the end for self-assessment.

1. What environmental factor is the primary cause of worsening COPD symptoms?

   A. Increased physical activity

   B. Air pollution

   C. Consumption of organic foods

D. Use of indoor heating

2. Which type of workplace exposure can lead to the development or exacerbation of COPD?

A. Ergonomic stress

B. Bright lighting

C. Dust and chemical fumes

D. Office noise

3. How does climate change impact respiratory health?

A. By decreasing airborne allergens

B. By improving air quality

C. By increasing the frequency of wildfires

D. By reducing the length of pollen seasons

4. Which strategy can mitigate the impact of poor air quality on COPD patients?

A. Increasing outdoor activities

B. Staying indoors with air purification during pollution events

C. Removing indoor plants

D. Using outdoor exercise equipment

5. The use of personal protective equipment (PPE) is recommended for workers exposed to:

A. Computer screens

B. High levels of dust and chemicals

C. Office paperwork

D. Ergonomic keyboards

6. Ground-level ozone and particulate matter are associated with:

A. Cleaner indoor air

B. Decreased COPD exacerbations

C. Worsening of COPD symptoms

D. Enhanced lung function

7. Wildfires contribute to COPD exacerbations through:

A. The production of clean air

B. Reduction of outdoor temperatures

C. Emission of smoke and particulates

D. Increased humidity levels

8. A preventive measure for COPD patients during heatwaves includes:

    A. Spending more time in direct sunlight

    B. Wearing heavy clothing

    C. Staying hydrated and remaining in cool environments

    D. Increasing physical exertion outdoors

9. Policies that promote cleaner air and reduce emissions are essential for:

    A. Worsening the greenhouse effect

    B. Increasing global temperatures

  C. Mitigating the impact of climate change on respiratory health

    D. Reducing the efficiency of solar panels

10. Healthcare preparedness for environmental events affecting COPD patients involves:

    A. Reducing availability of emergency services

    B. Planning for increased demand and supporting vulnerable populations

    C. Discouraging the use of air purifiers

    D. Promoting outdoor rehabilitation activities

Answers:

1. B. Air pollution

2. C. Dust and chemical fumes

3. C. By increasing the frequency of wildfires

4. B. Staying indoors with air purification during pollution events

5. B. High levels of dust and chemicals

6. C. Worsening of COPD symptoms

7. C. Emission of smoke and particulates

8. C. Staying hydrated and remaining in cool environments

9. C. Mitigating the impact of climate change on respiratory health

10. B. Planning for increased demand and supporting vulnerable populations

Chapter 14: Advocacy, Awareness, and Support Networks

14.1 Building a COPD Community

The Power of Community in COPD Care

Creating a supportive community for individuals with Chronic Obstructive Pulmonary Disease (COPD) is essential for enhancing the quality of life, promoting effective disease management, and fostering advocacy and awareness. A robust COPD community provides emotional support, shared knowledge, and collective advocacy to address the challenges faced by those living with the disease.

Components of a COPD Community

- **Support Groups:** Support groups, whether in-person or online, offer a platform for individuals with COPD to share experiences, coping strategies, and encouragement. These groups can provide a sense of belonging and reduce feelings of isolation.

- **Patient Advocacy Organizations:** Organizations dedicated to COPD advocacy work to raise awareness, influence health policy, and secure funding for research and patient support. They play a critical role in improving care and outcomes for the COPD population.

- **Educational Resources:** Access to reliable and up-to-date information about COPD management, treatment options, and lifestyle modifications is vital. Communities often facilitate education through workshops, seminars, and online content.

- **Healthcare Professionals:** Doctors, nurses, respiratory therapists, and other healthcare providers contribute to the community by offering expert advice, medical care, and support for self-management practices.

Benefits of a Strong COPD Community

- **Improved Disease Management:** Sharing knowledge and experiences can help individuals navigate the complexities of COPD management more effectively.

- **Emotional Support:** Connecting with others who understand the challenges of living with COPD can provide emotional relief and reduce the risk of depression and anxiety.

- **Advocacy and Awareness:** A united community can advocate more effectively for policy changes, improved care, and increased research funding, benefiting the wider COPD population.

- **Education and Empowerment:** Through educational initiatives, individuals can learn to better manage their condition, leading to improved health outcomes and quality of life.

Building and Engaging with a COPD Community

- **Participation in Support Groups:** Joining a COPD support group can be a starting point for engaging with the community and benefiting from shared experiences.

- **Involvement in Advocacy Efforts:** Getting involved in advocacy campaigns can help drive positive changes for the COPD community at large.

- **Utilization of Online Platforms:** Online forums, social media groups, and websites dedicated to COPD can provide valuable resources and connections without geographical limitations.

- **Collaboration with Healthcare Providers:** Working closely with healthcare professionals can ensure that community efforts are informed, relevant, and supportive of overall COPD care.

Conclusion

Building and engaging with a COPD community is a powerful way to support individuals living with the disease. Through shared experiences, advocacy, and access to resources, a strong community can significantly impact disease management, emotional well-being, and the broader fight against COPD.

14.2 Advocacy and Policy Change

Driving Improvements in COPD Care and Awareness

Advocacy plays a critical role in shaping policies that improve care, increase awareness, and foster research in Chronic Obstructive Pulmonary Disease (COPD). Through concerted efforts, advocates can influence public health priorities, secure funding for COPD programs, and ensure that patients' voices are heard in policy-making processes.

Key Areas of Advocacy for COPD

- **Increased Funding for Research:** Advocates work to secure more funding for COPD research to understand the disease better, develop new treatments, and ultimately find a cure.

- **Access to Care:** Ensuring that all individuals with COPD have access to high-quality healthcare, including diagnostic tools, medications, pulmonary rehabilitation, and support services.

- **Clean Air Legislation:** Promoting policies that reduce air pollution and protect lung health, such as stricter emissions standards for industries and vehicles, and regulations on tobacco use.

- **Public Awareness Campaigns:** Raising awareness about COPD, its risk factors, and the importance of early diagnosis can lead to earlier treatment and better outcomes for patients.

- **Workplace Protections:** Advocating for regulations that protect workers from exposure to respiratory hazards in the workplace, reducing the risk of occupational COPD.

Strategies for Effective Advocacy

- **Building Coalitions:** Collaborating with other health organizations, patient groups, and healthcare professionals can amplify the impact of advocacy efforts.

- **Engaging Policymakers:** Directly engaging with legislators and policymakers to educate them about COPD and the needs of patients can influence policy decisions.

- **Utilizing Media and Social Media:** Leveraging traditional and social media to raise awareness and rally public support for COPD-related policies and funding.

- **Empowering Patients:** Encouraging patients and their families to share their stories and experiences with COPD can personalize the disease's impact and motivate change.

Impact of Successful Advocacy

Successful advocacy can lead to significant improvements in COPD care and awareness, including:

- Enhanced funding for research and development of new treatments.

- Broader access to diagnostic and treatment services for patients.

- Stronger protections against air pollution and workplace hazards.

- Increased public and political awareness of COPD as a critical health issue.

Conclusion

Advocacy and policy change are vital for advancing the fight against COPD. By pushing for increased research funding, improved patient care, cleaner air, and greater disease awareness, advocates can help reduce the burden of COPD on individuals and society. Engaging in advocacy efforts empowers patients, families, and healthcare professionals to contribute to meaningful change and improve the lives of those affected by COPD.

14.3 Navigating Healthcare and Insurance

Overcoming Barriers in COPD Management

For individuals living with Chronic Obstructive Pulmonary Disease (COPD), navigating the complexities of healthcare systems and insurance coverage is a critical aspect of managing their condition. Ensuring access to necessary treatments, medications, and support services can significantly impact the effectiveness of COPD management and the patient's quality of life.

Key Challenges in Navigating Healthcare and Insurance

- **Coverage Variability:** Insurance plans vary widely in terms of what treatments and medications they cover, which can affect patients' access to the latest COPD therapies and rehabilitation programs.

- **Costs:** Even with insurance, the out-of-pocket costs for medications, pulmonary rehabilitation, and medical equipment (such as oxygen concentrators) can be prohibitively expensive for some patients.

- **Complexity of Healthcare Systems:** The complexity of healthcare systems can make it difficult for patients to understand their benefits, rights, and the processes for accessing care and submitting insurance claims.

Strategies for Navigating Healthcare and Insurance

- **Education and Advocacy:** Educating oneself about COPD, available treatments, and specific insurance plan details is crucial. Patients can also advocate for themselves by requesting coverage reviews or appealing denials for necessary treatments.

- **Utilizing Patient Assistance Programs:** Many pharmaceutical companies and nonprofit organizations offer patient assistance programs that provide medications at reduced cost or for free to those who qualify.

- **Seeking Support from Healthcare Providers:** Healthcare providers can be valuable allies in navigating insurance issues, as they can provide necessary documentation and support appeals for coverage of treatments and therapies.

- **Exploring Public and Community Resources:** Government programs and community-based organizations may offer additional support for individuals with COPD, including access to healthcare services, financial assistance, and social services.

The Role of Healthcare Providers in Patient Support

Healthcare providers can play a significant role in assisting patients with COPD to navigate healthcare and insurance challenges by:

- Providing clear information about the diagnosis, treatment options, and management strategies for COPD.

- Assisting with the documentation needed for insurance claims and appeals.

- Referring patients to patient assistance programs, public health programs, and community resources.

Conclusion

Navigating healthcare and insurance is a complex but essential part of managing COPD effectively. By becoming informed, advocating for themselves, and utilizing available resources, individuals with COPD can improve their access to necessary treatments and support services. Healthcare providers, patient advocacy groups, and support networks can offer valuable assistance in overcoming the barriers to effective COPD care.

14.4 Exercise: 10 MCQs with Answers at the End

Test your understanding of advocacy, awareness, support networks, healthcare navigation, and insurance challenges in COPD management with these multiple-choice questions. Answers are provided at the end for self-assessment.

1. What is a primary goal of COPD advocacy?

   A. To reduce public interest in COPD.

   B. To increase funding for COPD research and improve patient care.

   C. To limit access to COPD treatments.

   D. To discourage smoking cessation efforts.

2. How can support groups benefit individuals with COPD?

   A. By offering a platform for sharing experiences and coping strategies.

   B. By providing a cure for COPD.

   C. By eliminating the need for medical treatment.

   D. By increasing pollution levels.

3. Which strategy is effective in raising COPD awareness?

A. Ignoring symptoms of COPD.

B. Using social and traditional media for education and advocacy.

C. Discouraging the use of healthcare services.

D. Limiting discussions about COPD to medical professionals only.

4. A challenge in navigating healthcare and insurance for COPD includes:

A. Too much coverage for COPD treatments.

B. The simplicity of healthcare systems.

C. Variability in insurance coverage and costs.

D. The overabundance of affordable medications.

5. What role do healthcare providers play in supporting COPD patients' navigation of insurance issues?

A. Reducing the effectiveness of treatments.

B. Providing documentation and support for insurance appeals.

C. Discouraging the use of patient assistance programs.

D. Promoting self-management without professional guidance.

6. An effective method for COPD patients to manage healthcare costs is to:

A. Avoid seeking any medical advice.

B. Utilize patient assistance programs and explore public resources.

C. Increase out-of-pocket expenses.

D. Use only traditional remedies to treat COPD.

7. Advocacy efforts for COPD are aimed at:

A. Decreasing public awareness of the disease.

B. Increasing the cost of COPD care.

C. Promoting policies that protect lung health and improve patient care.

D. Discouraging research into new treatments.

8. COPD communities and support networks can help individuals by:

A. Isolating them from others with similar experiences.

B. Providing emotional support and shared knowledge.

C. Encouraging the discontinuation of treatments.

D. Increasing exposure to COPD triggers.

9. The complexity of healthcare systems affects COPD management by:

A. Making it easier to access the latest treatments.

B. Simplifying the process of insurance claims.

C. Making it difficult for patients to understand their benefits and rights.

D. Reducing the costs associated with COPD care.

10. Public health campaigns for COPD awareness are crucial for:

A. Discouraging early diagnosis and treatment.

B. Reducing knowledge about the disease.

C. Encouraging smoking and other harmful behaviors.

D. Promoting early diagnosis, treatment, and smoking cessation.

Answers:

1. B. To increase funding for COPD research and improve patient care.

2. A. By offering a platform for sharing experiences and coping strategies.

3. B. Using social and traditional media for education and advocacy.

4. C. Variability in insurance coverage and costs.

5. B. Providing documentation and support for insurance appeals.

6. B. Utilize patient assistance programs and explore public resources.

7. C. Promoting policies that protect lung health and improve patient care.

8. B. Providing emotional support and shared knowledge.

9. C. Making it difficult for patients to understand their benefits and rights.

10. D. Promoting early diagnosis, treatment, and smoking cessation.

Chapter 15: Living Well with COPD

15.1 Strategies for Daily Living and Independence

Living well with Chronic Obstructive Pulmonary Disease (COPD) involves adopting strategies that enhance daily living, maintain independence, and improve the overall quality of life. Managing COPD is not only about medical treatments but also about making lifestyle adjustments and adopting practices that help individuals navigate the challenges of the disease more effectively.

Key Strategies for Enhancing Daily Living with COPD

- **Energy Conservation:** Learning to conserve energy can help individuals with COPD minimize fatigue. This includes planning activities, taking regular breaks, and using labor-saving devices.

- **Breathing Techniques:** Practicing breathing techniques, such as pursed-lip breathing and diaphragmatic breathing, can help manage breathlessness during activities.

- **Exercise and Physical Activity:** Regular, moderate exercise improves cardiovascular health, muscle strength, and endurance. Pulmonary rehabilitation programs offer tailored exercise routines that are safe and beneficial for people with COPD.

- **Healthy Diet:** A balanced diet rich in fruits, vegetables, lean proteins, and whole grains can help maintain a healthy weight, improve energy levels, and support overall lung health.

- **Quitting Smoking:** Smoking cessation is the most effective step for slowing the progression of COPD and improving lung function.

- **Stress Management:** Managing stress through relaxation techniques, mindfulness, and hobbies can improve mental health and enhance coping mechanisms.

- **Avoiding Triggers:** Identifying and avoiding triggers, such as air pollution, cold air, and allergens, can help prevent exacerbations and improve daily comfort.

- **Regular Medical Check-ups:** Keeping up with regular medical appointments and following the treatment plan, including taking medications as prescribed, are crucial for managing COPD effectively.

- **Home Modifications:** Simple home modifications, such as removing rugs to prevent falls, installing grab bars in the bathroom, and ensuring good indoor air quality, can make daily living safer and more comfortable.

- **Social Support:** Staying connected with family, friends, and support groups provides emotional support and can help individuals with COPD maintain a positive outlook.

Empowerment Through Education

Education plays a vital role in living well with COPD. Understanding the disease, its triggers, and management strategies empowers patients to take an active role in their care. Healthcare providers should offer educational resources and guidance to help individuals with COPD make informed decisions about their health and lifestyle.

Conclusion

Living well with COPD requires a comprehensive approach that includes medical treatment, lifestyle adjustments, and proactive management strategies. By adopting practices that enhance daily living and independence, individuals with COPD can lead fulfilling lives despite the challenges of the disease. Collaboration with healthcare providers, support from loved ones, and engagement with the COPD community are key components of successful disease management.

15.2 Nutrition and Exercise: A Holistic Approach

Optimizing COPD Management Through Diet and Physical Activity

A holistic approach to managing Chronic Obstructive Pulmonary Disease (COPD) emphasizes the importance of nutrition and exercise as foundational elements of overall health and well-being. Proper diet and regular physical activity can significantly impact lung function, symptom management, and quality of life for individuals with COPD.

Nutrition for COPD: Fueling the Body

A balanced diet supports lung health, provides energy, and helps maintain an optimal weight, which is crucial for managing COPD symptoms and preventing exacerbations.

- **High-Quality Proteins:** Essential for repairing and building muscle, including the respiratory muscles. Sources include lean meats, fish, eggs, dairy, and legumes.

- **Complex Carbohydrates:** Provide sustained energy. Whole grains, fruits, and vegetables also offer vitamins, minerals, and fiber that support overall health.

- **Healthy Fats:** Omega-3 fatty acids, found in fish, nuts, and seeds, have anti-inflammatory properties beneficial for lung health.

- **Antioxidants:** Vitamins C and E, found in a variety of fruits and vegetables, can help reduce lung inflammation and protect against cell damage.

- **Adequate Hydration:** Staying well-hydrated helps thin mucus, making it easier to clear from the lungs.

Exercise: Enhancing Lung and Overall Health

Physical activity is essential for strengthening the muscles used in breathing, improving circulation, and enhancing the body's use of oxygen.

- **Pulmonary Rehabilitation:** Offers a supervised, comprehensive exercise program tailored to individuals with COPD, focusing on improving endurance and respiratory muscle strength.

- **Walking:** A low-impact activity that can be easily adjusted to fit individual fitness levels and capabilities.

- **Strength Training:** Builds muscle strength, including the respiratory muscles, improving daily function and independence.

- **Flexibility and Balance Exercises:** Yoga and tai chi can improve flexibility, reduce stress, and enhance balance, reducing the risk of falls.

Integrating Nutrition and Exercise

Adopting a holistic approach involves integrating nutrition and exercise into daily routines:

- **Consult Healthcare Providers:** Before starting any new exercise regimen or making significant dietary changes, consult with healthcare professionals to ensure safety and appropriateness.

- **Set Realistic Goals:** Start slowly and gradually increase intensity and duration to build stamina without causing undue fatigue or exacerbations.

- **Monitor Progress and Adjust as Needed:** Regularly evaluate how diet and exercise are affecting COPD symptoms and overall health, adjusting as necessary to continue making positive strides.

Conclusion

A holistic approach to COPD management, incorporating balanced nutrition and regular exercise, can significantly improve lung function, reduce symptoms, and enhance quality of life. By working closely with healthcare providers and adopting sustainable lifestyle changes, individuals with COPD can lead healthier, more active lives.

15.3 Mental Health and Emotional Well-being

Addressing the Psychological Aspects of COPD

The impact of Chronic Obstructive Pulmonary Disease (COPD) extends beyond physical symptoms to include significant psychological and emotional challenges. Anxiety, depression, and feelings of isolation are common among individuals with COPD, affecting their quality of life and ability to manage the condition effectively. Addressing these mental health concerns is a crucial component of comprehensive COPD care.

Common Mental Health Challenges in COPD

- **Anxiety:** Worries about breathlessness, future health, and the ability to perform daily activities can lead to persistent anxiety.

- **Depression:** The chronic nature of COPD and the limitations it imposes can contribute to feelings of sadness, hopelessness, and loss of interest in enjoyable activities.

- **Social Isolation:** Physical limitations and fear of exacerbations may lead individuals to withdraw from social interactions, exacerbating feelings of loneliness.

Strategies for Supporting Mental Health and Emotional Well-being

- **Professional Support:** Seeking help from mental health professionals can provide effective strategies for managing anxiety and depression. Therapy, such as cognitive-behavioral therapy (CBT), and in some cases, medication, can be beneficial.

- **Support Groups:** Participating in COPD support groups, whether in person or online, allows individuals to connect with others facing similar challenges, share experiences, and offer mutual support.

- **Physical Activity:** Regular exercise, as part of a tailored pulmonary rehabilitation program, can improve mood, reduce anxiety, and enhance overall well-being.

- **Stress Management Techniques:** Practices such as mindfulness, meditation, and deep breathing exercises can help manage stress and promote relaxation.

- **Maintaining Social Connections:** Engaging in social activities, even if they need to be adapted to accommodate physical limitations, helps reduce feelings of isolation and supports emotional health.

- **Education and Empowerment:** Understanding COPD and being actively involved in treatment decisions can empower individuals, reduce anxiety about the condition, and improve coping skills.

The Role of Healthcare Providers

Healthcare providers play a key role in recognizing signs of mental health struggles in patients with COPD and providing or referring for appropriate support and treatment. Routine screening for anxiety and depression, along with discussions about emotional well-being, should be part of regular COPD care.

Conclusion

Mental health and emotional well-being are integral to living well with COPD. By acknowledging and addressing the psychological impacts of the disease, individuals with COPD can achieve better management of both their physical and emotional health. Support from healthcare professionals, mental health specialists, and the COPD community is vital for fostering resilience and enhancing the quality of life for those affected by COPD.

15.4 Exercise: 10 MCQs with Answers at the End

Test your understanding of living well with COPD, covering strategies for daily living, nutrition and exercise, mental health, and emotional well-being, with these multiple-choice questions. Answers are provided at the end for self-assessment.

1. What is crucial for conserving energy in daily activities for individuals with COPD?

   A. Avoiding all physical activities

   B. Planning and pacing activities

   C. Increasing caffeine intake

   D. Sleeping less

2. Which breathing technique can help manage breathlessness in COPD?

   A. Rapid shallow breathing

   B. Pursed-lip breathing

   C. Holding breath for long periods

   D. Breathing exclusively through the nose

3. Regular, moderate exercise for COPD patients can lead to:

   A. Decreased lung function

   B. Increased risk of exacerbations

   C. Improved cardiovascular health

   D. Higher dependency on oxygen therapy

4. A balanced diet for someone with COPD should NOT include:

   A. High-quality proteins

   B. An excess of processed sugars

   C. Healthy fats

   D. Antioxidants

5. Why is smoking cessation important in COPD management?

   A. It increases lung capacity instantly

   B. It slows the progression of the disease

   C. It eliminates the need for medication

   D. It improves the taste of food

6. Professional mental health support for COPD may involve:

   A. Cognitive-behavioral therapy

   B. Avoiding all social interactions

   C. Ignoring symptoms of depression

D. Increasing physical isolation

7. Support groups for COPD provide:

A. A platform for smoking cessation only

B. Financial compensation for participation

C. Opportunities to share experiences and coping strategies

D. A cure for COPD

8. Stress management techniques beneficial for COPD include:

A. High-intensity exercise

B. Mindfulness and meditation

C. Ignoring symptoms of stress

D. Avoiding all forms of relaxation

9. Maintaining social connections in COPD helps to combat:

A. Improved lung function

B. Social isolation and loneliness

C. The need for medication

D. The effectiveness of pulmonary rehabilitation

10. In managing COPD, healthcare providers play a key role in:

    A. Discouraging exercise and activity

    B. Recognizing and addressing mental health issues

    C. Recommending smoking as a stress reliever

    D. Increasing patients' dependency on healthcare systems

Answers:

1. B. Planning and pacing activities

2. B. Pursed-lip breathing

3. C. Improved cardiovascular health

4. B. An excess of processed sugars

5. B. It slows the progression of the disease

6. A. Cognitive-behavioral therapy

7. C. Opportunities to share experiences and coping strategies

8. B. Mindfulness and meditation

9. B. Social isolation and loneliness

10. B. Recognizing and addressing mental health issues

Conclusion

As we conclude our comprehensive journey through understanding Chronic Obstructive Pulmonary Disease (COPD), it's clear that managing this condition requires a multifaceted approach. From the basics of understanding COPD, through the complexities of its diagnosis, treatment strategies, and the impact of environmental and occupational factors, to the importance of advocacy, support networks, and living well with the disease, each aspect plays a vital role in enhancing care and improving the quality of life for individuals affected by COPD.

Key takeaways include:

- **Early Detection and Comprehensive Management:** Timely diagnosis and a holistic management plan that includes medical treatment, lifestyle adjustments, and regular monitoring are crucial.

- **Lifestyle Modifications:** Smoking cessation, a healthy diet, and regular exercise are fundamental to managing COPD effectively.

- **Mental Health and Emotional Support:** Addressing the psychological aspects of living with COPD is as important as managing the physical symptoms.

- **Community and Advocacy:** Engaging with support networks and participating in advocacy efforts can provide valuable resources and contribute to broader change in how COPD is perceived and treated.

- **Navigating Healthcare:** Understanding how to navigate healthcare systems and insurance, and advocating for access to necessary treatments and support, is essential for optimal COPD care.

- **Environmental Awareness:** Recognizing and mitigating the impact of air quality, occupational hazards, and climate change on lung health is critical for preventing COPD exacerbations and progression.

This exploration underscores the importance of education, empowerment, and proactive engagement for individuals living with COPD, their caregivers, and healthcare providers. Together, through informed decision-making, advocacy, and the implementation of effective management strategies, it is possible to face the challenges of COPD and work towards a better quality of life for those affected.

*The best way to thank an author
is
to write a review.*

9 789334 040333